The Doctor-Patient Relationship in Pharmacotherapy

Improving Treatment Effectiveness

The Doctor-Patient Relationship in Pharmacotherapy

Improving Treatment Effectiveness

Allan Tasman, MD

Michelle B. Riba, MD, MS

Kenneth R. Silk, MD

THE GUILFORD PRESS
New York   *London*

©2000 The Guilford Press
A Division of Guilford Publications, Inc.
72 Spring Street, New York, NY 10012
www.guilford.com

Printed in the United States of America

This book is printed on acid-free paper.

Last digit is print number: 9 8 7 6 5 4 3 2 1

Library of Congress Cataloging-in-Publication Data
Tasman, Allan, 1947–
    The doctor-patient relationship in pharmacotherapy : improving treatment effectiveness
/ Allan Tasman, Michelle B. Riba, Kenneth R. Silk.
        p.   cm.
Includes bibliographical references and index.
ISBN 1-57230-596-7 (cloth)
    1. Psychopharmacology.   2. Psychotherapist and patient.   3. Mental
illness—Chemotherapy.   I. Riba, Michelle B.   II. Silk, Kenneth R., 1944–   III. Title.
RC483.3 .T375 2000
616.89′18—dc21   00-037114

About the Authors

Allan Tasman, MD, is Professor and Chair in the Department of Psychiatry and Behavioral Sciences at the University of Louisville. He served as President of the American Psychiatric Association from 1999 to 2000. Dr. Tasman is a nationally known psychiatric educator, psychoanalyst, and cognitive neuroscience researcher. He has a long-standing interest in the clinical integration of biological, psychological, and psychosocial treatment approaches.

Michelle B. Riba, MD, MS, is Clinical Associate Professor and Associate Chair for Education and Academic Affairs in the Department of Psychiatry, University of Michigan, and is currently Secretary of the American Psychiatric Association. Dr. Riba is a consultation-liaison psychiatrist and Director of the Psycho-Oncology Program at the University of Michigan Comprehensive Cancer Center.

Kenneth R. Silk, MD, is Associate Professor and Associate Chair for Clinical and Administrative Affairs in the Department of Psychiatry and Chair, Faculty Group Practice Board, University of Michigan Health System. Dr. Silk is an active clinician and teacher whose research interests are in the area of personality disorders.

About the Contributors

James M. Ellison, MD, MPH, is Clinical Director of the Geriatric Psychiatry Service at McLean Hospital in Belmont, Massachusetts, and Associate Clinical Professor of Psychiatry at Harvard Medical School. Dr. Ellison maintains an active private and consulting practice. He has published on clinical psychopharmacology, emergency psychiatry, and the interface between psychotherapy and pharmacotherapy.

Michael D. Jibson, MD, PhD, is Clinical Associate Professor and Director of Residency Education in the Department of Psychiatry at the University of Michigan. Dr. Jibson's clinical and academic interests include phenomenology and clinical psychopharmacology of schizophrenia, assertive community treatment for severe mental illness, and psychiatry education.

Jonathan M. Metzl, MD, is a lecturer in the Department of Psychiatry and Assistant Research Scientist in the Women's Studies Program at the University of Michigan. Dr. Metzl is also Co-Director of the University of Michigan Interdisciplinary Institute. Dr. Metzl has published widely on the intersections between psychiatry, cultural studies, and the humanities, and is a nationally known expert on visual representation in psychotropic advertisements.

Preface

In recent decades there have been dramatic changes in the nature of psychopharmacology practice in psychiatry. Several factors account for these changes. First, tremendous advances in neuroscience have led to increased sophistication in our development of new medications for the treatment of psychiatric illnesses. New medications, an explosion of research regarding medication treatments, and the development of protocols involving simultaneous use of several medications have all contributed to this growth. We are more sophisticated and effective than ever in the pharmacologic interventions we make with our patients.

Unfortunately, our increased sophistication in psychopharmacology has been influenced negatively by the wave of managed care that has swept the United States. Because of reimbursement policies, managed care programs, in a misdirected attempt to reduce the cost of psychiatric treatment, have forced many psychiatrists to alter inappropriately their practice patterns.

These changes have led to the widespread use of the 15-minute "medication check" as a primary treatment intervention. Contrary to everything we have learned regarding the importance of a biopsychosocial approach to patient care, medication prescription in this treatment approach has been separated from psychotherapeutic or psychosocial interventions. Often, the psychiatrist's role is limited to medication prescription, and other treatment interventions are provided by other mental health clinicians. It is almost always the case that there is less than optimal contact between the psychiatrist and the other clinicians providing care. This has led to a situation in which at least one large managed care firm has demonstrated that the costs of providing treatment in this model are actually higher than in a model wherein psychotherapeutic and psychopharmacologic care is provided by the psychiatrist.

The impact of these managed care changes on psychiatric education has also been an unfortunate one. Training programs throughout the United States have de-emphasized psychotherapy training and decreased curriculum time devoted to helping residents learn the subtleties of the interpersonal relationships involved in any type of treatment intervention. Many psychiatrists who have graduated from residency programs in the past decade, or who are now in training, have not had adequate opportunities during residency to understand the way the doctor-patient relationship can be used effectively as the context for all psychiatric treatment, especially regarding pharmacologic interventions.

We have written this book in an attempt to provide psychiatrists with this important body of information that may have been inadequately addressed during their training. It is well known that treatment outcomes are improved when the treatment interventions are made within the context of a trusting, caring, and ongoing relationship with a clinician. Compliance problems with treatment are a major cause of poor treatment outcome, especially when the treatment is primarily pharmacologic. Thus, the ability to monitor and use the relationship between the physician and the patient to improve compliance is essential. A patient's sense of well-being, resulting from a respectful interpersonal relationship, provides a synergistic effect to the desired pharmacologic effects of treatment. Every psychiatrist can benefit from attention to these issues, especially in the present treatment environment.

It has been a pleasure to work in collaboration with Michelle Riba and Ken Silk on this text. In addition, our other collaborators, Drs. Ellison, Jibson, and Metzl, have been outstanding contributors with whom to work. Thanks also go to Linda Gacioch in Michelle Riba's office, who provided all of the logistic support for this project. Finally, particular thanks go to Kitty Moore, our editor at The Guilford Press. Kitty's initial enthusiasm for this project provided an impetus for our undertaking it. In addition, her helpful comments and facilitative approach have helped us produce a work that is superior to what might have been produced without her assistance.

We feel confident that our readers will find this book as enjoyable to read as it was to produce, and that the information contained here will lead to better clinical care.

ALLAN TASMAN

Contents

CHAPTER ONE

Overview and Framework

Case 1

Mr. A, a 47-year-old married male who worked in the financial industry had been suffering with bipolar disorder for about 15 years. It had been very difficult to stabilize him on medications, and over the years he had vacillated between being depressed and lethargic to being hypomanic and ultimately frankly manic. His mania led him to psychotic thinking, and he ended up telling his bosses at work how to run the company. Eventually, he lost his job and was hospitalized. He moved back home from another state and had been my patient for only 6 weeks. I had seen him for four sessions, an hour intake and three half-hour "med checks." In my initial assessment, I felt that he had finally attained some sort of stability since his last hospitalization 6 months before. Thus I was surprised when I received a call from our emergency room stating that Mr. A was there with his wife. He was quite hypomanic and was refusing medications. I asked the worker in the emergency room if she would put Mr. A on the phone.

> Dr. A: How are you doing?
> Mr. A: Great, just great, Doc. How are you?
> Dr. A: Well, I am a bit worried about you. The folks in the emergency room think you are a bit "up there" (*a chuckle from the patient*), and that has me worried, especially since they say you don't want to take any medication.
> Mr. A: That's not true, Doc. I am happy to take my lithium. I

just don't want to take that Risperdal again. You know how groggy it makes me.

DR. A: I know, but I am worried that this is going to lead to your going in the hospital again, and I know how much you hate that. Do me a favor, will you? Would you take that Risperdal now, and I'll see you first thing in the morning and we can go from there and figure things out. But I want you to take the medication before you leave the emergency room.

MR. A: OK, Doc. Sure. I'll see you in the morning, but you better tell my wife what time the appointment is, because I don't think I'll remember it.

DR. A: Sure, and thanks.

MR. A: No problem, doc. See ya'.

Most psychiatrists today prescribe medications and, for many, the focus of their practice is on offering psychotropic treatment. Busy clinicians may have only 20 minutes with a patient to prescribe, monitor, and initiate changes in the medication regimen. In such a brief amount of time, what role can the doctor-patient relationship play in a psychiatrist's work, particularly in prescribing? Evidence shows that without a solid doctor-patient relationship, many treatments can be potentially derailed. As the case of Mr. A shows, this patient would have been much less likely to cooperate with the emergency room clinician's suggestions and much less likely to respond to his psychiatrist's advice without a doctor-patient relationship. In this book, we hope to show how even in the current medication-focused environment, the doctor-patient relationship can be quite substantial and have a critical impact on the clinical course and outcome of treatment.

As we all know, how we practice psychiatry has changed dramatically with biological psychiatry, molecular biology, and managed care. Yet the foundation of psychiatry still remains rooted in the doctor-patient relationship. We see the doctor-patient relationship as one of the essential features that defines the practice of psychiatry, and we will try to show how the doctor-patient relationship pervades and remains the support structure of every aspect of the practice of psychiatry.

This chapter will briefly discuss issues and topics related to the doctor-patient relationship that will be covered in more detail in the chapters that follow. This chapter will cover issues such as how the doctor-patient relationship can affect the course of illness, how the relationship can enhance adherence (as suggested in the opening example), as well as how it can encourage the patient to be open to discussing his reactions to medication with his physician. In addition, we explore how the doctor-patient relationship can enhance the effects of medications. And finally, we suggest that the positive relationship that develops between patient and physician can serve as a model upon which other relationships for the patient can be built or modified.

This book will remind us that even as psychiatry grows more scientific, it is not merely a science, but an art as well. If we can attend to and develop the art, the beneficial effects of the science may flourish even more.

PSYCHIATRY AND THE DOCTOR-PATIENT RELATIONSHIP

Given today's current healthcare climate, the idea that we even have time for a relationship with our patients is frequently questioned. Questions range from whether the doctor-patient relationship is useful or necessary, to the more sophisticated inquiry as to whether it is cost effective. Few would deny the usefulness of a "positive" feeling between any patient and her physician, yet the question does arise as to whether the extra time and energy required to fully develop a doctor-patient relationship adds any value to the treatment. In other words, is what you get for the extra time and effort to establish and enhance a positive relationship worth the time (and therefore the money) that it consumes to accomplish it? To determine cost effectiveness, we can look at how the relationship matters when we are assigned the role primarily of a psychopharmacologist.

Obviously, a key aspect of psychopharmacology is appropriate diagnosis and treatment with the right medications. Yet ensuring that the medications are taken is equally important. The process of diagnosis as well as the process of ensuring compliance with medications can be accomplished more smoothly, successfully, and safely when the clinician attends to and conveys to a patient an interest in who she is, her daily life, and how the medication affects different aspects of her life. Compliance with the medication regimen is essential to a reasonable outcome in many psychiatric cases, and a mutually respectful doctor-patient relationship can only enhance compliance. Without gathering information about the patient and the patient's behavior in the past, the psychopharmacologist cannot predict adherence to a treatment regimen. Moreover, the manner

3

and attitudes of the psychopharmacologist during the process of gathering that information has a profound effect on the nature of the doctor-patient relationship.

The following case illustrates how failing to gather even basic information, such as how the patient had gotten to the hospital (driven himself) and how far he lived from the hospital, led to the patient being prescribed increasing dosages of medication which affected his ability to get himself safely home. There could have been a very problematic and even deadly outcome if the outpatient therapist, who knew the patient well, had not listened to the patient and intervened. Further, the patient's overwhelming lethargic response to the medication certainly would almost guarantee noncompliance once the patient left the hospital.

Case 2

Mr. B is a 35-year-old middle manager who was admitted to the hospital in a suicidal state. One of the stressors contributing to his increasing depression was his poor relationship with his wife. In fact, his wife refused to drive him the 25 miles to the hospital on the morning of admission even though he expressed suicidal ideation and the fleeting idea of running his car into a bridge abutment. He was passive in light of what he considered to be somewhat abusive but certainly dismissive behavior by his wife, and he felt that in the hospital he was just as unable to assert himself as at home. He remained in the hospital for 5 days during which time substantial doses of an additional antidepressant and a sleeping medication were added to his already preexisting complicated regimen of psychotropic medications. He had orthostatic hypotension, and he felt spacey, dizzy, and at times confused. His bedtime sleeping medication had been increased until he slept through the night, though he said he had told his treating psychiatrist that his sleep was always terrible in the hospital and sleep was not a major concern to him before he came into the hospital. Fortunately his outpatient therapist came to see him on the day designated for his discharge, and noticing his lethargic and hypotensive state requested that the "new" medications be held for a day so that the patient could drive himself home. The treating inpatient psychiatrist seemed unaware of the fact that the patient had to drive himself home and appeared to have ignored the patient's statement that he always slept poorly while in the hospital. Further, it seemed much safer for the patient to make that drive midday one or two days later rather than during early evening rush hour with the sun low in the horizon, the time originally scheduled for the discharge.

The failure of the inpatient psychiatrist to listen to the patient and to take what he said seriously could have had disastrous consequences for the patient if he had had to drive home in his somewhat drowsy state. The inability of the inpatient psychiatrist to even realize the extent of the patient's lethargy reveals the psychiatrist's adherence to a medication regimen over a patient's stated set of feelings and needs. Recall that the patient did not feel that he had to sleep well while in the hospital; yet the psychiatrist kept increasing the medication dosage to get him to sleep leading to a possible discharge of a lethargic and inattentive-to-task individual.

ESTABLISHING AN INTERPERSONAL FRAMEWORK THROUGH THE DISCUSSION OF MEDICATIONS

In the process of prescribing, there are many different ways in which we can try to convey to the patient our interest in what it is like for him or her to take the medication, and by extension an interest in how the patient feels about life in general. Conveying this interest begins during the initial prescribing time, generally during the initial appointment. Some of the ways that interest can be conveyed are (1) presenting who you are and what it is you believe as a physician-psychiatrist, (2) psychoeducation, (3) dialogue, (4) emphasizing choice, and (5) reiterating that you want to know how the patient feels, both good and bad, about and after taking the medications. Underlying each of these types of interactions are empathy on the part of the psychiatrist as well as patience in allowing the patient to speak and express how he feels or what he is trying to say. In other words, prescribing medications gives us the opportunity to emphasize our interest in how taking the medication impacts upon the patient's life and how the patient deals with the positive effects as well as the side effects. It provides an arena where the patient will be encouraged to turn to the psychopharmacologist for more help along the way should it be necessary.

Patients come to us with many preconceived ideas; some ideas are about the psychiatrist himself and some are about the benefits or dangers of medications. Some patients are shackled with the shame that they are unable to get better without chemicals, and some with the thought that

5

once the chemicals are finally straightened out, everything will be fine and life will suddenly go back to how it was before they became ill. All of these preconceptions will have an effect on how they respond to the psychiatrist and to the medication regimen, as well as on the patient's daily life.

How can we make use of attitudes about medications to enhance the development of the doctor-patient relationship? Take, for example, the many patients who arrive in your office claiming they have what they think is a chemical imbalance. These patients obviously have a preconceived notion about how their disorder developed and may well assume that any medication will redress this imbalance, restoring their lives to their previous states. While evidence points to the fact that chemicals mediate all our emotions, thoughts, movements, and behaviors, we rarely know exactly the balance of environmental and neurochemical factors. Was it an environmental stressor that brought about the imbalance or the chemical imbalance and the lack of stress tolerance with subsequent symptom formation? From our perspective, it is critical that the patient understand that "chemical imbalance" explains only part of the picture. Without sitting down with the patient and providing information about how mental disorders develop, the patient will not have the opportunity to appreciate his role as well as his resources in the development, maintenance, or remission of certain symptoms. The techniques employed in the following clinical vignette involve two issues: (1) presenting who you are and what it is you believe as a physician-psychiatrist, and (2) psychoeducation (i.e., the way one can usefully appreciate the role of biochemicals in symptom formation or maintenance).

Case 3

Ms. C: Hello, Doctor. My primary care physician sent me over to you to get some antidepressants. I have been having many symptoms of depression for many years, and he says that it is all in my chemicals, that I have a chemical imbalance, and all I need is some medication.

Dr. C: Well, let's get a history of what has been going on with you. [The history and other relevant information are taken, and the psychiatrist is prepared to prescribe and does prescribe medication.] While I think that the medications will prove to be quite helpful to you, I want to say something about medications and chemical imbalance. It is true that chemicals probably underlie and mediate all our thoughts, moods, and feelings, and it is also true that some people believe that medications correct those imbalances and people then just get better. I am not a fan of that particular explanation, because it doesn't seem to give you credit for the things you might do to make the depression and your life better. We psychiatrists still do not know the relationship between stress and the chemical changes that take place with stress, though there is much work going on in that area. Nonetheless, I think it sells you short and ultimately might make you feel more helpless and hopeless if the medications don't get you completely better, because then it would mean that there was nothing that you could do to make things better. So I want to pay attention not only to how the medication is making you feel, as well as to the side effects of the medication, but I also want us to think about things such as how you are doing overall, how things are going along with your husband and kids, how your job is going, and any other thing that you think impacts upon how you might be feeling at any time. OK?

Ms. C: OK. But I think it will be a waste of time because I think I just need to get my chemicals in line.

Dr. C: Well, we will have 30 minutes [or 15 minutes] when we meet, and checking on the medication and its side effects should take about 5 minutes, so if you don't mind, I will try to ask you questions about these other things because I think getting to know you should make everything go a little more smoothly.

In this case, the psychiatrist made clear that her interest lay not only in finding the right medication but in making sure the patient understands her perspective on depression and its treatment. From the very beginning, she shows her interest in the patient's reaction to taking medication (3-5 above) and in ensuring the patient finds the treatment process collaborative. In that initial appointment, and after discussing the medication or medication choices and the possible side effects attendant to each, we might say:

"If something strange happens or you get a bunch of weird feelings even if they are things that I haven't mentioned today, I want you to give me a call. Don't assume that it's nothing, because perhaps it might really be something, and any individual person may have a unique response to a given medication. Even if a side effect is very rare and may not be mentioned on the medication sheet [which we give to each patient], if you get the side effect, for you it's not rare at all; in fact it's 100%. On the one hand, I don't want you to automatically decide that it's the medication, and then you stop taking it; nor do I want you to assume it's nothing when it might truly be related to the medication. There are many different medications [for depression, confused thoughts, mood swings, etc.], and there is no need for you to have to suffer through a side effect that may be particular to one medication when there are others on the shelf that we could use. So if you feel strange or 'antsy' or whatever, give me a call and we can talk about it and decide together where to go from there."

Many clinicians balk at suggesting to patients "the phone lines are always open." Yet in our experience, very few patients take us up on contacting us outside of office hours. In addition, greater availability and interaction at the outset of treatment will probably pay extra dividends in more cooperation and success in the overall compliance with the medication. Patients who know they can call you and not be greeted by a hostile, off-putting response are more likely in the long run to tolerate greater amounts of discomfort. It is important to remember that the goal is to work with the patient so that he will take the medication and comply with the dosing schedule. What we are trying to establish at the outset is making sure the patient understands how the therapy is to work. It also shows the patient your interest as to how the patient is feeling; and it establishes an atmosphere in which the patient's feelings, worries, and concerns are serious and valid experiences worthy of discussion.

To take this process apart even further, I'll tease out the different elements that convey your interest in the patient as an individual and thus in the collaborative relationship between you and him.

- We repeatedly use the word *we* rather than *I* to imply that decisions and discussions are really going to be a mutual, cooperative, collaborative effort between the two of us (dialogue).
- We repeatedly make it clear we encourage the patient to tell us how he feels and reacts, and if he gets worried or concerned, you want to know about it ("If something strange happens . . . I want you to give me a call" [reiterating that you want to know how the patient feels, both good and bad, about and after taking the medications]).
- We validate that the patient's feelings and reactions are important ("Don't assume that it's nothing").
- We point out to the patient that you consider him to be an individual (". . . any individual person"), and that you will take the issue of his unique attitudes seriously (choice and individuality).

- It reinforces the idea that you think that taking some medication is important and would help but the medication does not have to be this particular medication ("There are many different medications" [choice]).
- It presents as well as models the circumstance that you and he will work jointly to solve problems (". . . we can talk about it and decide together" [dialogue and choice]).

MAINTAINING AN INTEREST IN INTERPERSONAL ISSUES

Opportunities will continue to arise during the course of treatment that will allow you to reinforce the collaborative approach to the treatment process. Each occasion should be used carefully to reassure the mutual respect and thus hopefully to enhance the patient's self-respect. These opportunities often occur around medication adjustment or change, particularly when the patient is having a side effect to the medication or when the medication appears to have lost its effectiveness. In this example, dialogue and choice are emphasized.

Case 4

Ms. D is a 32-year-old single professional woman with a family history of schizophrenia, though she herself appears to have suffered throughout her life with mild depression. She has suffered for many years with depressive episodes, one severe enough to lead her to miss 8 weeks of work. She takes citalopram (40 mg), and she was doing well on that for 6 months before becoming moderately (not enough to stay home from work) depressed. Previously, she had done well for four months on 20 mg of citalopram, and the citalopram was increased 6 months ago because she then also had a breakthrough of moderate depressive symptoms. The question was whether to increase her citalopram to 50 mg or 60 mg, to switch her to another antidepressant, or to perhaps augment her regimen with buproprion. She was in psychotherapy with a social worker at the same agency where Dr. D worked.

Dr. D: Let me go over the choices I think we have. First we could do nothing, but I think you have been struggling with this increasing depression for 3 weeks, so I think we would both feel better by doing something. We can either increase the citalopram or change to another antidepressant or add another drug.

Ms. D: Well, I would prefer not adding another drug if we could do something else.

Dr. D: Well, my inclination also is to stick with and increase the citalopram. Let me tell you why. To change to another drug would probably mean, depending on the drug chosen, taking you off citalopram and waiting [if the other medication also increased serotonin] about 10 days before starting the new drug; and then we have a 3-week wait to see if the new drug is working better. If we increase the citalopram right now, we know you tolerate the side effects well, and we will perhaps know sooner whether the increase has worked.

Ms. D: I don't mind just increasing the medication, but I am concerned that it will work for a while and then not work. We have twice had this happen, first when the citalopram was at 20 mg, and now when it is at 40 mg. What will we do then?

Dr. D: Well, we'll be in the same boat we are in now except that I would probably switch you then or add another medication, though I know you are concerned about too many medications. So I guess we would switch, and let me remind you that there are many antidepressants available to us.

Ms. D: That's OK with me. Let's increase it, but if it works and then fades again, I do want to get off it. You know, every time I get depressed, I am fearful of getting so depressed I will have to stop working again, and I don't think I or my employer could tolerate that happening again. And even if they keep me on, they will probably not see me as very reliable and stop giving me important and interesting assignments.

Dr. D: I agree. My goal is to have you remain not depressed. Fortunately, this time you are not so depressed that you can't work, so certainly the medications are at least helping to maintain a level where you can do things, not with great *joie de vivre*, but with enough ability to maintain attention and concentration. But I know this isn't good enough for you for the long run.

Ms. D: You are right about that. Now if I increase to 60 mg, I will need a prescription today because I will run out before next week.

The interchange reveals a number of different things about the interpersonal relationship between the patient and the prescribing psychiatrist. In this particular case, the patient was also in a "split treatment" because she was in psychotherapy with a social worker. Even though she is getting psychotherapy elsewhere, her appointment with the psychopharmacologist also deals with psychological issues beyond medication management. The psychiatrist is aware of the patient's concern about being able to keep working, and she takes this into consideration when exploring a change in medication ("I am fearful of getting so depressed I will have to stop working again"). Further, the psychiatrist is aware that the patient expects a high level of quality of work from herself ("But I know this isn't good enough for you in the long run"). And the psychiatrist acknowledges that she and the patient want the same outcome ("My goal is to have you remain not depressed").

There are a number of items in this interchange that reinforce the general interpersonal issues we are trying to emphasize. The psychiatrist uses the word "we." The psychiatrist "thinks out loud" and tries to provide the patient with some sort of choice ("Let me go over the choices I think we have"), and to let her react to the choice. This is not done in a completely passive way because the psychiatrist certainly has an opinion, but the psychiatrist's opinion is presented in the spirit of dialogue rather than dictum (". . . my inclination is to . . ."). This perhaps facilitates the patient expressing her worries ("I am fearful of getting so depressed I will have to stop working again"), and the psychiatrist acknowledges the worries and tries to give an opinion on how the thing she is worried about will be addressed in the future (". . . I know this isn't good enough for you for the long run").

Once again, we see in this example that the patient feels comfortable that her concern about the symptoms will be considered seriously by the psychiatrist in determining whether or not the medication should be changed. By being treated as an informed consumer, she has a say in her treatment that can only translate into a sense of control of the outcome. She can also, in the process of being told her choices, be reassured that she is not at the end of the line with regard to treatment choices (". . . let me remind you that there are many antidepressants available to us"). It also models the idea that things are not just black or white or right or wrong, that is, that there are choices and options in most of what we do in life. Modeling of interpersonal behavior in the office can be carried out into interpersonal situations in the rest of the patient's social relationships.

MEDICATION ADHERENCE AND SYNERGISM
WITH THE DOCTOR-PATIENT RELATIONSHIP

As we have pointed out, there are a number of positive benefits from such a collaborative approach. Indeed, we can point specifically to some of these benefits. First, a collaborative approach reassures the patient that he won't have to fight with you to discuss the possibility of discontinuing a medication that has been quite intolerable for him. Perhaps he is weakened by depression and worried about holding his job. Fighting with you can only deplete him further. An open attitude assures him that his needs will be given careful consideration. Second, the knowledge that you want to hear how he is really feeling may help him to tolerate early side effects. He has firsthand evidence that he won't have to bear side effects that are too severe or endure them for too long a period. In addition, one cannot overlook the placebo effect of medications. While there is no specific understanding as to why the placebo effect occurs, issues such as physician faith that the medication will work, patient's desire to please a physician whom he likes, and the charisma (and perhaps renown) of the physician may all play a role in the effect (Brown, 1998).

In the era before the advent of the newer antidepressants and the newer atypical antipsychotics, commonly used medications had side-effect profiles that caused more difficulty in a greater percentage of patients than our newer compounds. For example, the tricyclic antidepressants (TCAs) almost universally caused dry mouth that persisted as long as the patient was on the medication (Bassuk & Schoonover, 1978). The TCAs also had a strong predilection for causing constipation, and many people felt "hung over" with a mild to moderate frontal headache (Remick, 1988). Patients had to be convinced to remain on the medications for the three weeks or so that it took for them to finally begin to feel as if the medications were working. As far as the patient was concerned, in the beginning weeks after initiating the treatment, the cost and inconvenience of the side effects far outweighed any therapeutic benefit that she was experiencing. Thus frequent telephone contacts and exhortations to stick with the medication were necessary until the benefits of the medication could be more readily experienced. Yet, even after the patient had a therapeutic and beneficial response to a TCA, the side effects remained troublesome to many patients, and a good doctor-patient relationship was needed to keep the patient willing to endure the uncomfortable aspects of the medication in order to benefit from its positive therapeutic effects.

Contrast this to many patients' experiences with the selective serotonin reuptake inhibitors (SSRIs). Most patients who do not experience sexual side effects from these compounds are reluctant to stop taking these medications! The SSRIs are quite effective for most people, and most patients experience minimal side effects and many feel no side effects whatsoever. Perhaps the "easier" side-effect profile of the newer class of psychotropic medications may make it seem, then, at first glance, less necessary to develop and maintain a solid doctor-patient relationship (Feighner, 1999; Steffens et al., 1997). In some cases, this may indeed be true. For those patients who respond immediately to medications, they may not need the same level of care. And yet, as this book will show, a solid doctor-patient relationship has an effect from the very first meeting in regard to compliance, response to side effects, and so forth, even with patients who respond well to medications.

When the doctor values the interaction with the patient, the response to side effects will be less intrusive. If you have ever felt unappreciated, undervalued, or simply irritated, you might have discovered your tolerance level for minor insults drops. Considering that our patients are, at the outset, beset with feelings of anxiety, depression, insecurity, and loss of self-esteem, we can appreciate that they might find even the most minor of side effects annoying and disruptive. If, however, in their interactions with us, our patients feel positive about themselves, then these patients may be able to increase their tolerance of some of the uncomfortable side effects that accompany almost any psychotropic medication regimen.

Further, if the patient experiences each and every visit to us as irritating, frustrating, or belittling, then one can predict the effects of those encounters downstream. The patient will avoid appointments in whatever way possible. Some patients will grow passive when they come to see you. Others will simply stop taking the medication and thus avoid seeing you at all. Others will take the opposite approach, by making a lot of noise. Perhaps they will complain about each and every side effect, or about the lack of rapidity of therapeutic change, or give you a host of other nonspecific complaints. You may find yourself wondering if the patient is simply trying to drive you crazy or get attention. Perhaps she is, but it may be that she is trying to tell you she doesn't feel heard or valued. These transference-countertransference issue are discussed in Chapter 5 in this book.

If we set the tone of good listeners, we can create a situation where the patient will feel safe enough to talk about some of the more annoying side effects of medications. For example, many patients are reluctant to talk about sexual concerns that can arise with SSRIs. They don't want to explore their personal sexual activity with you and yet it may be that this side effect is very disturbing to them. Unless there is a feeling in the office of genuine interest in the quality and variety of the patient's life activities and experience, the topic may not come up even if the psychiatrist asks directly about sexual interest. We may find the patient replying "It's OK," even when worries, concerns, and actual performance problems are occurring, and the patient may have a good deal of anxiety about the effects of this change in interest and behavior on his or her partner. Ultimately a failure in the interpersonal relationship between doctor and patient to set a mood wherein such topics are discussed will lead to noncompliance or irregular compliance with the medication. Or the patient may not get the full benefit of the medication because despite being much less depressed, he is worried and sad about his loss of sexual functioning or reactivity.

It is not unusual for patients to feel "weak" or "morally lax" if they are told that they need to take medications. Unless we show an interest in what they think about their having to take medications, we may lose an important variable that can have repercussions in treatment and compliance. In addition, patients have other worries about medications, some of which they may not address because they feel foolish or too anergic, or too low in their own self-esteem to really believe that what they think or care about has any importance. Some of these issues, questions, or worries that our patients may have relate to whether or not the medication is addicting, whether or not they can really feel sad (should the occasion arise) when they are taking, for example, antidepressant medication, and what other people will think about the medications. Certainly not all patients bring these issues up and the issues may not be important or relevant to many patients. Some of these concerns are more subtle and complicated than those that directly deal with side effects. These concerns may reflect the patient's general attitude toward any medication or may involve the patient's thoughts about how people they live with view the idea of psychiatric medication. If we miss important clues, we may end up with a patient who unpredictably doesn't take his medication, as the following case shows.

Case 5

Mr. E, a 33-year-old married insurance salesman, presented with all the classic symptoms of major depression. He had been struggling with depression his whole life but was reluctant to take medications for fear that they would make him too happy and thus not very considerate of other people in his life, and that they would be addicting.

MR. E: But, Doc, I can't keep going on like this.

DR. E: Let me tell you how I think about antidepressant medication. I do not think it makes you so happy that you walk around all day with a grin on your face. Rather, I think of them as providing a kind of safety net for you. Now when you get depressed, you seem to crash down through the whole house and wind up in the dank, dark basement. Antidepressants keep you from falling below the first floor. You will still get sad when it's appropriate, you will still be able to show genuine concern for other people, and hopefully you will be able to experience a fuller range of positive and negative feelings. These feelings will be "safer" for you to experience. Also, while these medications are not addicting, people can experience an increase in symptoms if they stop them too suddenly. But if we are careful and do a slow taper when you wish to stop them or when we both feel it is time to stop them, there should be a minimal amount of difficulty. We just need to work together, and you need to keep me informed of your worries and concerns so we can together decide how to proceed if and when these problems occur.

INFORMATION SHARING AND PRIVACY ISSUES

There are other people in the patient's life with whom our relationship plays an important role in the ultimate outcome of the treatment process. First, there is the issue of managing split treatment wherein the psychotherapy or case management is being provided by one person and the medication by another (Riba & Balon, 1999). In these instances, the interpersonal relationship between the two individuals involved in the treatment plays a crucial role in how the patient views and experiences each aspect of the treatment. Certainly if there is not mutual respect between the different providers, then the division between the clinicians may be exploited by the patient and/or acted out by the providers (Gross-Doehrman, 1976), even without their realizing what they are doing. The first step is for both parties to understand what each specialist can provide. Unrealistic expectations can lead to straining the relationship between the patient and either or both of the providers (Silk, 1999). In the most complicated situations, a provider attempting to live up to unrealistic expectations can lead to a kind of therapeutic heroism and enthusiasm that often can evolve into complex and perhaps uncomfortable, innovative biological and psychotherapeutic regimens and combinations (Main, 1957). One of us recalls an analyst who admitted a very severe, primitive, and regressed patient with borderline personality disorder into the inpatient unit. When the unit director spoke with the referring analyst on the phone in order to determine what she thought was needed from the hospitalization, the analyst replied, most seriously, "Fix her and get her to stop cutting." You can appreciate how complicated such a situation can be when such is the therapist's expectation and this expectation, most assuredly, had been conveyed to the patient in some manner or form.

This reasoning can also be extended into consideration of the relationship between the psychopharmacologist and the referring primary care physician, or the spouse or parents or other members of the family. Certainly, as mentioned above, if there are serious sexual side effects, the patient's partner may be less than supportive of the patient taking medication, and may thus subtly or not so subtly undercut compliance with the medication regimen. Even if the patient is aware of the fact that there may be many alternate choices among a given class of psychotropics, the patient's spouse may be unaware that such flexibility exists. Or the spouse may be embarrassed that the patient is taking medication, or pass some moral judgment on the patient. Or a boss may wish to speak with the psychopharmacologist about the effect of the medication upon the patient's ability to perform tasks at work, such as operating dangerous machinery.

The arena gets even more crowded as we add other providers, both medical and nonmedical, as well as family members or employers or teachers, to the situation. What does it mean to think about our interpersonal relationship with these people who populate the patient's life? How will our speaking to or at least our reacting to requests made upon us to speak to all these people impact upon the patient and the patient's sense of privacy and of being an important, unique individual, as was emphasized at the beginning of this chapter? Again, a decent, positive, collaborative, working relationship with the patient will help mitigate any serious difficulties that could occur around the issue of sharing information with others. If a relationship of mutual discussion and problem solving has been established since the beginning of treatment, then these issues are approached in the spirit of mutual problem solving. For example, the clinician can talk with the patient about what she thinks she would need to tell his boss about how the medication might affect the patient, and together decide how to best approach her. Or the clinician can ask the patient the best way to communicate with her spouse to make clear that the side effects might mitigate over time, or the decision to change medications if they do not.

Sharing of information with others involved with the patient may take on a different tone if one is doing primarily psychotherapy rather than psychopharmacology with the patient, but for our purposes here, let us consider only the psychopharmacologic treatment. What the psychopharmacologist is often able to share with significant or important "others" involved with the patient are the facts of the psychopharmacologic (i.e., purely psychiatric) treatment. These are issues related to diagnosis, medication treatment, choice of medication, side effects, ultimate prognosis, and so forth, and these are not issues related to what one might label *content* or *process* issues in the treatment. Though content or process issues might seem to occur more readily in a more purely psychotherapeutic treatment, recall that we are emphasizing that a relationship, and then by definition these types of process/content interpersonal issues, occur in all types of treatment. If a relationship of mutual discussion and problem solving has been established since the beginning of treatment, then a dialogue as to who is to be spoken with, how the request was made, and what is to be shared, can begin. Matters such as whether the patient will be or wants to be present during the discussion with other people need to be raised. The psychopharmacologist can review beforehand what it is that she plans to share with the significant other, while allowing the patient to question, to veto, and to elaborate upon some of the issues or topics that are suggested as possible points of information or discussion. At the conclusion of the discussion about talking with another person, the physician then asks the patient if there is anything that she or he specifically does not want to be shared, and also anything that the patient specifically wants shared. Further, there needs to be an assurance that if the meeting with the other person occurs when the patient is not present, then the psychopharmacologist will review at the next scheduled session with the patient what was said during the meeting with the other person. If there is no appointment scheduled for a number of months, we suggest an extra appointment not only so that the patient knows what was discussed, but also to avoid having the patient building up some fantasy about what was discussed at the meeting with the other person. Remember that our interest here is to do all we can to maintain an open, positive, interactive doctor-patient relationship.

Case 6

Dr. F: I got a call from your manager, and she was wondering how you were doing, and I said that I wanted to talk with you first. I know she knows you are seeing me because you went to her when you got worried and depressed, and she referred you to me. But before I talk with her, I want to know if there are things you think she should or shouldn't know. Then I would want to tell you what I would tell her, and have you react to that so we can come to some agreement on what I will be saying, and you will know what was discussed between her and me. Of course you can be present, or if it is decided that we speak by telephone, you can be on another phone so you can be involved in the discussion. Or if it doesn't work out that way, I'll review with you my discussion with her when you and I meet next Wednesday. OK? Any questions or concerns?

Not only will discussions rather than dictums around these kinds of issues continue to foster a relationship of mutual discussion, problem solving, and respect, they also model for the patient how interpersonal relationships can be conducted with the goal of mutual respect and problem solving. It allows an opportunity to model how two people can overcome possible differences or disagreements, how two people can learn to listen and perhaps modify each of their opinions upon listening to someone else's point of view, and how two people form compromises and follow through upon them.

Case 7

Dr. G: You know, when I first brought up the idea that your boss wanted to talk with me, all you could say is "no." You even threatened to go see someone else if I didn't stop talking about it. I suggested that I would be willing to hear your viewpoint if you would be willing to hear mine, and we did that and we just had a meeting with your boss. She assured you that they were behind you all the way. In fact she even told us about her sister who also had depression. So you and I were able to listen to each other and then decide whether and how to have the meeting. You know, sometimes I think your initial reaction and response here happens with you in other circumstances as well, that is, that you decide something and you don't want to hear anyone else's opinion about it. I think, if you want, you might find it useful to discuss this with Dr. H, your therapist, during your appointment with him next week. If you do, I would appreciate hearing what the discussion was like.

Thus another benefit of considering, developing, and paying attention to the relationship between oneself as physician and the patient is that it can serve as a model upon which other relationships can be built or modified. This is not an unimportant aspect of any treatment, particularly since many of our patients have disturbed interpersonal relationships, frequently as a secondary consequence of their disorder, though at other times perhaps as the primary stressor that may have been a significant precipitating contributor to the current episode. Whatever the circumstance or the relationship of the interpersonal difficulty to the present psychiatric situation, there is clear evidence from a number of studies that interpersonal stressors can help bring forth or help maintain current psychiatric difficulties (Kendler et al., 1999). By extension, then, the ability to cope with or to make interpersonal events less stressful might contribute to a substantial reduction in the intensity or frequency of future exacerbations of episodes of illness (see Table 1.1).

CONCLUSION

In this area of rapid treatment with its myopic focus on the particular effect of a given medication upon a given molecular structure or neurotransmitter or chemical reaction as part of a sophisticated cascade of molecular-biological events, we must pause and reflect on what it is that makes psychiatry special. The unique aspect of psychiatry comes from its psychological approach to the patient's life. Whether or not you are focused on a biological disorder, the impact of the disorder on all aspects of the patient's functioning will have an impact on the course and outcome of the disorder. In addition, psychiatry must never stop considering how the patient feels about having a psychiatric disorder or at least about having been labeled with a psychiatric disorder. As psychiatrists, we must not forget that the most important thing(s) in most people's lives are their relationships to other people. When we enter into the process of providing treatment to another person, we enter into the world of interpersonal re-

TABLE 1.1. Establishing and Enhancing the Interpersonal Relationship in Medication Prescribing

1. Remember that a major tenet of the profession of psychiatry is appreciating and understanding the doctor-patient relationship.

2. At the initial appointment, make clear that you want to know things about them that go beyond their symptoms or their specific diagnosis. This involves scheduling enough time during the initial appointment so that some interchange beyond matters relating merely to symptoms and diagnosis can occur.

3. Inform patients that you are interested in more than whether or not they have a "chemical imbalance."

4. Reinforce the idea that the patient is an individual with individual responsivity, both in terms of effectiveness as well as side effects to the medications.

5. When actually prescribing medications, let patients know that you are available between sessions to discuss their worries, concerns, and side effects.

6. When actually prescribing medications, attempt to clarify the realistic and unrealistic aspects of the patient's expectations of the effectiveness of the medications.

7. When actually prescribing medications, let the patient know that there are other medications to choose from should this one not work out, and use this discussion to enhance the idea of collaboration.

8. When issues relating to whether information about the facts of the prescribing process need to be shared with other physicians, family members, employers, or others, discuss the process and solicit the patient's input on what can and cannot be discussed as well as the format and venue for the discussion.

9. Whenever possible during the prescribing process, use the pronoun *we* rather than *I*.

10. Keep in mind that the type of interpersonal relationship created in the office setting can be a model for the patient for interpersonal relationships in other areas of his or her life.

11. Remember that in almost every interaction, you have the opportunity to (a) present who you are and what it is you believe as a physician-psychiatrist, (b) provide psychoeducation that can dispel myths, (c) create dialogue, (d) emphasize choice, and (e) reiterate that you want to know how the patient feels, both good and bad, about and after taking the medications.

lationships. How we conduct ourselves in that regard, and how we consider and reflect upon and participate in that interpersonal relationship, not only can have a powerful impact on the person and the illness, but also may serve as a model for the patient for his or her own relationships.

This chapter has touched on a number of issues related to the importance in considering and keeping "live" on one's radar screen the measurement of the course of the interpersonal doctor-patient relationship in the practice of psychopharmacologic management. But a final point needs to be made. One cannot force oneself to be interested in patients or interested in the relationship between oneself and a patient. Such an attitude or posture comes from a number of different places. The first needs to be a genuine respect and appreciation of others. The second comes from learning to tolerate and appreciate the feelings and dilemmas that our patients present us with, and from maintaining an attitude on our part that our patients are not malingerers or ne'er-do-wells or lazy or troublemakers. Rather they are people who are doing the best they can, whatever that represents, in circumstances that are particularly difficult and stressful *for them.* All these latter points simply drive us to consider who is the person, apart from the disease, who sits across from us in our office. Such consideration, combined with the underlying premise of respect and appreciation of others, cannot lead to any place other than thoughtfulness about our relationships with other people, patients or otherwise.

Decades ago, most psychiatric residents were expected to enter into some personal psychotherapy. With the changes that have occurred in psychiatry that deemphasize psychotherapy for our patients, we seem to have lost the idea that psychotherapy or psychological treatment for ourselves might be useful. While we do not suggest that such an expectation be reinstituted with respect to psychiatric training, we do suggest that every psychiatrist, every mental health practitioner for that matter, should examine whether she or he holds and practices mutual respect and appreciation of others as individuals. Do we possess the ability to sit with and tolerate the very difficult feelings that others as well as we, ourselves, may possess?

Thus there are a number of reasons why we should pay attention to the interpersonal relationship even when our contact with the patient is limited to medication management or maintenance. The first is probably the most important and fundamental—the hallmark of our profession is that we study interpersonal relationships, and even the current emphasis on biological mechanisms and pathophysiology should not distract us from that fundamental tenet of the profession of psychiatry. The second is that of considering each encounter as an interpersonal interaction between two individuals. The third is that the establishment early in treatment of an atmosphere of mutual respect and collaboration enhances the probability that future difficulties can be dealt with through open and respectful discussion. Such discussion can lead to increased compliance with agreed-upon medical regimens, to fewer complaints about side effects of medications, and to an enhanced feeling of well-being that comes from a respectful interpersonal relationship, a feeling of well-being that can be synergistic to the desired effects of the pharmacologic treatment. And fourth, such discussion can become a model for the patient for other interpersonal situations, and then may, in turn, reduce interpersonal and other life stressors that may, under particular circumstances, impact upon the course of psychiatric illness (Table 1.2).

In "The Retreat from Patients" (1971) Kubie makes the distinction between being a psychiatrist and learning the facts of psychiatry and the process of becoming a psychiatrist. One can *be* a psychiatrist by accumulating all the requisite knowledge necessary to treat in an efficient medical manner all those patients who present to us with *bona fide* psychiatric diagnoses. It does not take particular skill or empathy to learn the specifics of prescribing medications and which medication to prescribe. But Kubie emphasizes that merely using, even successfully, that knowledge base

TABLE 1.2. Advantages to Considering the Doctor-Patient Relationship in Medication Prescribing

1. Increases respect patients have for our profession and increases our respect and understanding of them.
2. Builds a foundation upon which difficulties or concerns about medication and the prescribing process can be openly discussed.
3. Leads to increased compliance because it encourages dialogue between physician and patient.
4. Builds the patient's self-esteem, which can enhance the beneficial effects of the medication and strengthen the patient's ability to tolerate side effects.
5. Provides a model of interpersonal behavior that can be translated to other interpersonal situations for the patient.
6. Reduces the overall stress the patient feels when coming to appointments for medication prescription and maintenance, and thus reduces the overall stress in the patient's life.

with patients does not lead to our *becoming* a psychiatrist, even though we may, for all intents and purposes, actually be a psychiatrist. Kubie argues that only by sitting with, struggling with, and bearing the feelings, expressions, ambivalences, contempts, pains, and prides of our patients, in the service of building and maintaining an interpersonal (i.e., doctor-patient) relationship can we truly *become* a psychiatrist. It appears to us that what is unique about the practice of psychiatry is the art of our interest in and attention to building and enhancing the doctor-patient relationship while we endeavor to practice in a kind, intelligent, and evidence-based manner the more purely scientific aspects of our profession.

CHAPTER TWO

Forming an Effective Therapeutic Alliance

Jonathan M. Metzl, MD

Case 1

As always, Dr. F is running 20 minutes late. Harried and over-booked, he simply never seems to have enough time to meet all of the demands of his working day. As he enters the examination room to meet with his patient Gina B, he is already thinking about the many other patients lined up to see him.

Gina B is a 36-year-old book editor who returns to the clinic on her second visit after beginning treatment with Prozac.

"So how are the medications working?" Dr. F asks while flipping through the medical chart.

"Not so well," Gina B responds. "I'm still feeling quite down. And I think Prozac is making me feel nauseated. Maybe Prozac won't help me."

"Not at all," Dr. F explains. "Today's medications are highly effective—they just take a bit of time to work. And often the side effects dissipate in a few weeks. Why don't we increase your dose? You'll feel better in no time. I'll call the pharmacy for you—the prescription will be waiting for you by the end of the day."

"Thank you, Doctor F."

"Not at all."

Dr. F then moves on to the next patient.

This chapter takes a closer look at the therapeutic alliance in a prescription interaction. It might seem as if the intersubjective relationship between a patient and a prescribing psychiatrist is of secondary importance when medications are involved. Yet if one considers the interaction of Gina B and her psychiatrist, it is easy to see how the dismissive attitude of Dr. F is unlikely to make Gina feel comfortable about his recommendations, even if they are medically correct. Medications can become the primary focus of a consultation, and the focal agents of therapy. To cite the case above, medications are frequently discussed as "working" on problems, and "helping" bring about cures. Medications are thought of as having "efficacy" and "potency," thus subtly relegating their prescribers to the role of conduits. In the process, the participants in a clinical interaction can end up focusing upon their relationships with medication and not with each other. Physicians prescribe while patients ingest. The implication of such a construction is that medications do the work so that humans do not have to. In other words, talking and listening to each other are no longer deemed important if we are already talking and listening to Prozac.

Yet the value and usefulness of medications is diminished if not considered in the context of the relationship between patient and doctor. To be sure, medications which help patients feel better can help bolster this alliance by providing palliation and relief. Yet such benefits need to be viewed as components of a larger, human conversation, rather than being conversations in and of themselves.

Why is it important to pay attention to the therapeutic connection between doctor and patient? In the book *The Patient's Story*, Robert C. Smith argues that the therapeutic relationship is "a fundamental detention of care; this relationship should be monitored as closely and continuously as the temperature, the blood pressure, and the pulse rate of the patient" (Smith, 1996, p. 151). Indeed, the therapeutic bond between a prescribing physician and a patient can affect the more denotative aspects of psychopharmacological care, such as adherence (see Chapter 5) and follow-up. This bond can also affect the more connotative aspects of care, such as the respect, trust, and comfort experienced by patient and physician alike. A strong bond between doctor and patient enhances the chance of a successful outcome, and provides the foundation from which complications—in the way of untoward effects, nonresponse, and so forth—can be negotiated. In correlational investigations, the emotional bond between patient and caregiver has been shown to be a predictor of therapeutic success. The "helping alliance" has been shown to correlate positively with initial accurate therapeutic interventions, and in psychotherapy this alliance has been argued to contribute to outcome to the same degree as theoretic approach or the use of specific clinical techniques (Crits-Christoph et al., 1993; Luborsky et al., 1985). Patients who feel "understood and satisfied" in an initial interview are far more likely to return for a second visit (Zisook et al., 1978–79). Conversely, misalliances have been linked to early termination from psychotherapy (Magnavita, 1993). Finally, poor and infrequent communications between doctor and patient have been linked with outcomes ranging from patient dissatisfaction to increased probability of legal action (Riba & Balon, 1999). Together, these findings speak to the importance of paying attention to the therapeutic bond in even the most impersonal clinical encounters and warn of the dangers when the reciprocity of information exchange is not closely minded.

In the following section of this chapter I briefly define the therapeutic alliance, or more appropriately the therapeutic collaboration, and discuss its importance to the clinical interaction. Subsequently I divide what might be considered threats to the alliance—points where communication between patient and physician can break down—into four categories: factors that emanate from the patient; factors that emanate from the physician; factors presented by the system of care; and factors embedded in the culture within which the system is situated. These four categories will help us better understand the components of the psychopharmacological interaction. Rather than providing an exhaustive compilation, these categories allow for a means of conceptualizing, and then observing, the ways often-assumed aspects of a therapeutic relationship can work to impede the formation of a close bond between doctors and patients. Strategies for enhancing communication are then presented at the end of each section.

THE THERAPEUTIC ALLIANCE
IN A PRESCRIBING CONTEXT

The notion of the "therapeutic alliance" once implied a very specific type of power relationship. In early psychoanalytic thought, for example, clear demarcations of information exchange were constructed between patients and doctors (Freud, 1913). It was believed that patients spoke with very little conscious awareness of what they were saying. Doctors, meanwhile, listened, understood, and ultimately interpreted. Contemporary theorists, however, are much more likely to describe the therapeutic alliance as a *collaboration* in which both doctor and patient contribute (Hatcher & Barends, 1996). Here collaboration is meant to imply both the work and relationship aspects of the therapeutic situation, as well as the ongoing *process* of negotiation and mutual adjustment that takes place between two individuals in a clinical setting.

This latter definition is quite useful when thinking about the interaction surrounding the activity of prescription writing that occurs in contemporary medical culture. To be sure, doctors maintain a high degree of power over the treatment process (see the section on the physician, below). Patients, however, are far from passive supplicants. Rather they are ever-increasingly active participants in the process, empowered through means such as consumer choice of providers, and increasing information about medications available on television, in popular magazines, or on the Internet. As these changes in medical and popular cultures evolve, models that involve mutually negotiated decisions and solutions are far more likely to be effective.

And yet as many clinicians realize, attention to the therapeutic alliance can feel like the least valued aspect of the treatment process. Treatment sessions grow ever shorter, while the amount of time between office visits grows ever longer. Many patients are seen by alternate caregivers. There hardly seems time, let alone impetus, for the introspection required for alliance formation. My implicit argument in the remainder of this chapter, however, will be that physicians need to pay attention to the small details of their interaction specifically because of—or in spite of—these obstacles.

THE COMPONENTS OF AN EFFECTIVE THERAPEUTIC RELATIONSHIP

What type of therapeutic relationship is most conducive to the effective exchange of information? While generalizations are often difficult—each patient, and thus each clinical situation, calls for a different set of relational strategies—contemporary psychotherapy provides a series of relational guidelines based on the notion of *intersubjective discourse*. The notion of *intersubjectivity*, implying a two-way conversation between mutually respectful individuals, serves as a helpful concept for the prescribing clinician attempting to envisage a meaningful and successful interaction with a patient. To be sure, there are aspects of a prescription interaction that are unique, and make it quite unlike psychotherapy in important ways. (The complicating factors unique to psychopharmacology will be discussed in the sections that follow.) And yet much like psychotherapy, the psychopharmacology interaction is at its core a negotiation between two persons in a room. As such, a clinician should always keep in mind that the most meaningful interactions are ones in which both parties are involved in a mutually constructed and empowering dialogue. A patient will be more likely to feel like an active participant if he or she is involved in the decision-making process, rather than being "told what to do" by a physician, as if by decree.

Let us briefly consider a few of the important *models of intersubjective alliance formation* between patient and doctor that have been described by controlled outcome studies of psychotherapeutic clinical relationships. These models provide useful guidelines when considering a psychopharmacology interaction as well. For example, Morgan et al.'s (1982) outcomes study assessed therapeutic bonds between clinicians and patients using the Penn Helping Alliance Rating Method. Their findings, with medication interactions in mind, identify a series of relational characteristics believed to offer significantly better outcomes, as compared with dyadic interactions that do not demonstrate these characteristics. Morgan et al. describe the essential features of psychotherapy that offer maximal outcomes as divided into two types of clinical relationships, each of which illuminates important aspects of the intersubjective therapeutic collaboration (Tables 2.1 and 2.2). Using this division, we might consider several important caveats and strategies for a prescription interaction. I will discuss these and other caveats in greater length below.

Often in medication treatment, modes of clinical discussion can attribute numerous relational factors to medications, ranging from improvement to deepened connection between patient and clinician. A patient might relate a brightened affect by saying, "The Zoloft is helping me. Can you refill my prescription over the phone next time? I'm incredibly busy at work, and it's tough for me to come in sometimes." Similarly, in Case 1, Gina B's symptoms are described as having arisen "because of Prozac." While this might well be true, the discursive effect moves the discussion away from the process in the room, and away from the therapeutic collaboration. Further, such discussions can circumvent or displace discussions about the nature of the clinician-patient bond.

TABLE 2.1. Type 1: Helping Alliance

Type 1 is a helping alliance that depends on the patient's experiencing the clinician as warm, helpful and supportive. Key features include:

1. The patient feels that the clinician is *warm and supportive.*
2. The patient feels the clinician is helping in the *common goals of insight and improvement* (without indicating that his or her own efforts and abilities have gone into his or her own change).
3. The patient feels *changed* by the treatment, for example, describing himself or herself as "improved" or "less anxious."
4. The patient feels a rapport with the therapist; the patient feels *understood and accepted.*
5. The patient feels that the therapist *respects and values* him or her.
6. The patient conveys a belief in the *value of the treatment process* in helping him or her to overcome problems.

TABLE 2.2. Type 2: Working Alliance

Type 2 is a working alliance based on the sense of working together in a joint struggle against what is impeding the patient. The emphasis is on shared responsibility for working out the treatment goals and on the patient's ability to feel in partnership with the clinician.

1. The patient experiences himself or herself as *working together* in a joint effort, as part of a team, with the clinician.
2. The patient shares *similar conceptions* about the etiology of his or her problems.
3. The patient expresses the belief that he or she is *increasingly able to cooperate* with the clinician in terms of understanding his or her behavior.

The patient actually demonstrates abilities similar to those of the clinician, especially with regard to the tools for understanding. (This sign begins to show the development of a capacity to do for himself or herself without the clinician, i.e., autonomously, what they did together.)

Source: Morgan et al. (1982).

TABLE 2.3. Common Unrecognized Feelings and Resulting Behaviors in a Single Clinical Interview in Students, Residents, and Fellows

---

Unrecognized feelings elicited after a clinical interview

Common

Fears of losing control, addressing psychological material, appearing unpleasant, harming the patient

Unique personal issues (e.g., reminds one of own difficult divorce)

Performance anxiety

Uncommon

Sexual feelings, attitude favoring biomedical data, anger, fear of involvement, intimidation by patient, inadequacy, disdain

Identification with the patient

Unrecognized behaviors observed during a patient interview

Common

Overcontrol of the patient and interview (e.g., inappropriate interrupting or changing subject)

Avoidance of psychological material (e.g., death, loneliness, disability)

Superficial behavior (e.g., overly reassuring, overly social)

Passivity (e.g., no control or direction, inactive, detached)

Uncommon

Seductiveness

Critical, intimidating, passive-aggressive

Lack of respect and sensitivity

Withdrawal, distancing

Source: Smith (1996, p. 155).

Strategies. Using a supportive framework, a clinician can relate a patient's description of medication effects to point out examples of intersubjective process. For example, instead of taking the patient's claims of improvement at face value, the clinician might ask the patient to think a bit more about the meaning of his or her improvement. "I'm pleased that you are feeling better. Now that it might not seem as painful, do you have any further insight into what may have been causing you to feel so bad before?" Or similarly, "Can you tell me how you feel different? Now that you feel better, what do you think are reasonable goals for our interaction?" Highlighting process often enriches the therapeutic bond, and deepens a patient's understanding of the process of treatment.

After a patient has an established psychopharmacological treatment regimen, the relationships between doctor and patient can deteriorate into discursive patterns of supply and demand. Patients can "request" medications, while clinicians "call in" prescriptions long after the clinical interaction has ended, a point illustrated in the case example at the beginning of this chapter. These kinds of exchanges can leave the patient feeling like he or she is "following doctor's orders" instead of contributing to a mutually respectful relationship.

Strategies. When appropriate, clinicians should engage patients in a process of mutual decision making. A clinician can instruct a patient about strategies for dealing with commonly encountered problems even before they might occur. Somewhat similarly, a clinician can set an end point of treatment, and provide a patient with the skills with which to reach it. For example, when raising a patient's dose of medication, a clinician might say:

> "Nausea or irritability are common side effects. When these occur, I usually tell patients to increase the dose a bit more slowly—since patients seem to know their own response patterns. Our goal should be to get you to 40 mg within 2 weeks, but I think you are a better judge than I am about how quickly this jump should occur. Why don't you try to titrate your dose upwards over the coming days, keeping an eye on these effects. I'll leave it up to you to decide when to jump from 20 to 30 to 40 mg, depending upon your response. Call me if there are problems—but if not we can meet in a few weeks to see how you are doing."

WHAT COMPLICATES THE THERAPEUTIC ALLIANCE BETWEEN PATIENT AND PHYSICIAN

In the following sections I focus upon strategies for recognizing the ways in which communication can break down when medications are the topic of conversation between patient and physician.

To cultivate a working alliance, clinicians must learn to be keenly aware of the complications that can arise in the clinical encounter, and specifically of the barriers that can stand in the way of the formation of a successful connection. The remainder of the chapter will organize the more common complicating factors in the prescriptive relationship into four sections: complications arising from the patient, from the physician, from the medical system, and from culture. Each section then concludes with a discussion of strategies for dealing with these difficulties.

The Patient

An understanding of a patient's resistance to interpersonal connection has long been considered a staple of psychiatric treatment. In the context of a medication evaluation, resistance might imply several possible etiologies. For example:

Case 2

Josh M is a 21-year-old computer programmer referred for psychiatric evaluation by his primary care provider. The consultation note explains that Josh "has been increasingly socially isolated and withdrawn, and has refused treatment with an antidepressant medication." In the initial session of treatment, Josh M appears self-absorbed and defensive, explaining that "I am only here because I have to be." Throughout the course of the interview, he makes numerous negative references to psychiatrists as "head shrinkers and control freaks." The patient appears otherwise competent. He demonstrates no signs of psychosis or mania, but appears moderately depressed. However, Josh M demonstrates great difficulty answering what he describes as "feeling questions"—questions regarding his emotional state. He describes his mood as "fine," and is unable to elaborate further. When the discussion turns to medication treatment, he becomes markedly upset, and claims "You can't make me take anything."

When the Symptoms Limit Communication

It is of course vitally important to realize that many psychiatric illnesses can make communication between patient and physician exceedingly difficult. Sometimes patients resist involvement because of the nature of their illness. In Case 2, for example, a young male patient with early signs of schizophrenia might well demonstrate a high degree of suspicion toward the physician. Such symptoms might be quite difficult to discern, since patients can have great stakes in keeping their perceptions private. Moreover, privacy can be a requisite component of the disease. Symptoms such as impulsivity, delusions, or hallucinations can be major impediments to the clinical dialogue.

A far more subtle level of impairment is seen in patients with mild to moderate depression—certainly another possibility raised by Case 2. Depressed persons can present as irritable, anhedonic, or dejected. Meanwhile anxiety disorders—another potential diagnosis with Josh M—can cause reticence and withdrawal, as patients develop avoidant or defensive coping strategies for dealing with symptoms that are often as confusing as they are troubling.

For patients who suffer from these and other maladies, symptoms such as hopelessness, anhedonia, and poor self-esteem render the first-person narrative—as in "I am in pain," or "I am in need of help"—exceedingly difficult. In these examples and in many others, the effects of Axis I and Axis II diagnoses are made manifest by their effects upon interpersonal connection. Patients seem unable to connect, or to describe important aspects of their physical or emotional states of being. Or just as often, patients give subtle nonverbal cues—lack of direct eye contact or guarded body language, for example—that they feel uncomfortable or unable to enter into a therapeutic collaboration.

Simply stated, any communication difficulties stemming from the symptoms of illness can limit the possibilities of forming a strong alliance. As such, a thorough history and mental status examination are requisite components of treatment. The process can be difficult with patients such as Josh M, whose defensiveness and suspicion stand in the way of connecting with the clinician. Further complicating matters are a patient's expectations when referred for medications by another clinician. As Josh M would claim in the interview, "I don't see why you're asking so many questions. Didn't my doctor tell you which medications you should give me?"

I will discuss these complications at greater length below.

Psychodynamic Conflicts

Core elements of pharmacological treatment, such as the ability to follow instructions or the ability to describe side effects, can be obstructed by long-term characterological or psychodynamic conflicts, in addition to the difficulties caused by the cognitive effects of a given Axis I diagnosis, explained above. Such conflicts can specifically stand in the way of a psychiatrist's efforts to form a working relationship with a patient. For example, Josh M's resistance to medications might indicate larger issues—a sense of entitlement, a fragile sense of self, a need for control, or competition with authority—that are likely also manifest in other aspects of his life. This is not to say that entitlement, competition, or other psychodynamic issues should be treated with medications. Rather, a clinician must realize that medication can become symbols through which these issues can be acted out. Further, a clinician must try to remain cognizant of these conflicts when deciding upon the nature and type of interventions he or she will offer.

For example, a patient's feelings of competition with authority can be expressed through his resistance not only to the physician, but also to the medications the physician prescribed. Often, medications provide a more than convenient vehicle upon which such resistance can take place. Such sentiments can often extend well beyond the actual clinical encounter. Seemingly minor details—a physician's name on a prescription bottle, or the "authoritarian" treatment regimen—can come to stand in for contested and difficult aspects of the clinical relationship, and can thus severely impede the formation of the alliance. This can then alter factors ranging from adherence to outcome.

Noncooperation

Finally it is important to realize that an outpatient clinical relationship, like any relationship, requires the contribution of both parties involved. Without continued effort, even the best intended interventions will be ineffective. To be sure, a great deal of the responsibility for such effort rests squarely upon the shoulders of the physician. However, it is important to realize that the patient shares responsibility in this clinical collaboration as well. Numerous research studies have shown that patients rated as making strong positive contributions to the therapeutic alliance had good outcomes in psychotherapy (Luborsky et al., 1985). Meanwhile, patients who entered a clinical relationship demonstrating "negative disposition to the treatment situation" and "intransigence to the therapist's efforts to shore up the alliance"—through behaviors ranging from hostility, to withdrawal, to noncooperation—were less likely to receive therapeutic bene-fit (Marziali et al., 1981). Such factors are equally salient in pharma-cotherapy as they are in "pure" psychotherapy, because both types of in-teraction can be experienced as alienating and impersonal by some patients. Many patients have preconceived skepticism regarding medica-tions, for example, as "addictions" or as "crutches." These feelings can be especially salient in the case of psychotropic medications which, despite advances in the destigmatization of mental illness, carry negative conno-tations for many patients.

Strategies. First and foremost, a clinician should focus upon getting the diagnosis right. If resistance to medication is a manifestation of an Axis I illness, appropriate measures should be taken to assure that the condi-tion is adequately addressed and treated. It is important to keep in mind, however, that even in the most extreme cases, the therapeutic relation-ship is not defined by the prescription of medication. Rather, the pre-scription of medication should always be thought of as a component of the therapeutic interaction.

Expectations, Reservations, and Resistance

As mentioned earlier, a fundamental goal of the psychoanalytic approach to the therapeutic alliance lay in helping a patient better understand his or her resistance to interaction, connection, and ultimately, intimacy. In the psychoanalytic consulting room, the analyst's function often involved providing an environment in which a patient felt safe to reveal his or her innermost thoughts, and occasionally pointing out patterns and insights that the patient did not realize. Though markedly different in tone and content, the role of the physician in the medication interaction might be thought of in a similar light. His or her aim should in part be the creation of a therapeutic environment in which a patient feels safe to explore his or her state of mind. Even if the encounter is brief, a clinician needs to ensure that a patient feels at liberty to express his or her feelings and re-actions. For example, people can have very different emotional reactions to medications. One person's "miracle cure" can be another person's source of shame, while what one patient thinks of as a statement of a physician's "caring" might to another patient connote a physician's lack of concern. As such, it is important for clinicians to appreciate the specifics of a patient's history and the nature of his or her interpersonal interactions, and to directly address each person's expectations and desires at the outset of treatment whenever possible. Importantly, this means understanding negative feelings and emotions as well. The physician should seek to address reservations and to listen as openly and as empathically as possible, even when a patient's assumptions about the role of medications might conflict with his or her own. Moreover, the physician should always seek to offer realistic, honest appraisal.

Strategies. The case of Josh M, for example, presents a clinician with several modes of action. While the patient's defensiveness might have been off-putting, it is important to realize that such posturing is also a form of communication. Were a clinician to answer such defensiveness with avoidant, or closed-ended questions—"Do you hear voices?" "Do you fear crowds?"—the result would likely be a reification of the communication gap between doctor and patient. Thus whenever possible (and of course within reasonable limits), the clinician should attempt to point out resistance, either through observation or through open-ended questions. Questions or observations such as "This situation seems difficult for you" or "It seems like you might have some negative feelings about doctors or medications" can allow patients to express their concerns rather than act them out. It is exceedingly important to provide an environment in which patients feel comfortable describing such emotions, ranging from hesitation about doctors to fears of medications, and that such feelings are validated rather than dismissed. In turn, clinicians can let patients into their own decision-making process—"What would you like to do? Dr. F, your primary care doctor, thinks you might benefit from medications, and you seem to hate the very idea. I'm feeling caught in the middle. Any suggestions?"—thereby forging a deeper alliance with the patient.

Power in the Relationship

An interaction in which one person diagnoses an illness in, and prescribes a medication for, another person, is inherently a power relationship. For example, the physician has the power of the knowledge of diagnoses and treatments. Moreover, he or she represents the power of the medical institution within which the clinical encounter takes place. Finally, the physician is sanctioned with the legal power with which to prescribe medications that are otherwise unavailable to consumers. The patient, meanwhile, tacitly acknowledges this authority by the seemingly simple acts of describing his or her symptoms, or even by taking medications.

Of course this power differential between doctor and patient is in many ways a requisite component of the clinical relationship. Patients often come to doctors seeking information that they do not have themselves. And it does not seem like much of a stretch to assert that in often-regressive times of illness, the power of the doctor can impart an important sense of reassurance. However, it is vital to realize that the power differential between physician and patient, if not realized and acknowledged, can also work to impede the therapeutic dialogue. This is an especially important consideration when medications are involved. The vignette in Case 2 provides an illustration of the ways in which the "power" represented by the doctor can also function as an obstacle to open communication. Patients referred by another provider might feel their very presence in a psychiatrist's office to be a position of disempowerment—as if their problems were "too crazy" to be handled by the referring doctor or therapist. Moreover, patients might also feel that a consultation with an "expert" means, a priori, that they will be required to begin psychopharmacological treatment.

Strategies. In this context, clinicians should attempt to subtly empower patients when possible and appropriate. As described above, clinicians can enlist patients in the decision-making process. Descriptions of treatment options should be presented in ways that allow patients to feel a sense of agency ("Several categories of medications might make you feel better. An antidepressant works by. . . . An anxiolytic works by. . . . What do you think would be the best course of action?"). Similarly, nonacute patients who voice reservations about medications can be asked to research medication options and diagnoses in the time between office visits, rather than to feel pressured about making an important decision on the spot ("It seems you have some reservations about this type of treatment. Would you like some time to learn more about the SSRI antidepressants, and then return to discuss this further?"). Suggestions might include speaking to friends who take the same medications, research on-line, or recommended first-person memoirs (Jameson, 1995). Finally, the clinician should continually seek a patient's input when changes in a treatment regimen occur, such as increasing dosage or switching medication.

Such strategies allow patient and clinician to collaborate in response to the patient's illness, rather than to independently seek to control it. The ultimate goal should be a sense of working together, through mutual responsibility. Open and honest discussion can enhance cooperation regarding the process of mental illness—a process that should privilege cooperation over compliance, and understanding over rote performance. To be sure, medications can empower patients by making them feel better. But interactions with a respected ally, a collaborator who values their opinion, can empower patients all the more.

Shame

Shame, like power, can also operate beneath the surface to impede communication. A growing body of literature has recently examined the ways in which positions long held as "therapeutic"—a doctor's reticence, for example, or a patient's requisite stance of pained revelation—can serve to censure the open and honest exchange of affect between clinician and patient. Broucek and Ricci (1998) discuss the importance of mutually realized needs in even the most highly prescribed clinical situations:

> If shame or shame anxiety are the principle affects regulating self-disclosure and communication, then it would seem that one of the aims of good technique should be to reduce the patient's shame and anxiety to levels more conducive to self-revelation. Intense shame can be so aversive, noxious, and self-fragmenting that the therapist may have to assist the patient in modulating it. Many patients will be helped by the identification and open discussion of their shame feelings; others will react with more shame to any attempt to directly address their shame. (p. 435)

These same tensions are often at play in a prescription interaction. Patients, for example, enter into examination rooms and are asked to relate deep, often highly personal aspects of their lives to a person who is often a complete stranger. Moreover, as I discuss below, the very fact that their primary care physician has implied that they may require treatments with "psychiatric medications," or has sent them to a psychiatrist for a consultation, can play upon long-held fears and assumptions. Such suggestions can be interpreted as an implication on the part of the physician that the patient's problems are too serious, or too threatening, for their interaction. Another unintended message might be that the physician does not want to hear the patient's problems, and is thus sending him or her elsewhere or attempting to silence a deeper discussion.

Strategies. Ricci uses "deshaming self-revelation" to describe voluntary self-disclosures designed to mitigate the isolation of a patient's shame (Broucek & Ricci, 1998). The term is meant to imply a strategy whereby a therapist presents himself or herself as someone who has experienced stressors similar to those presented by the patient, and survived. The therapist, in other words, subtly tells the patient that he or she is not alone, and that others—the clinician included—have realized similar feelings of isolation and despair.

To be sure, self-disclosure is a tangled web, and is not appropriate in all cases. Nonetheless, the strategy of limited self-disclosure is important to keep in mind. Perhaps a clinician has had similar reluctance to take medications, or has experienced untoward effects from a prescription, or has dealt with the difficulties of the medical system from the role of the patient. Phrases as simple as "I know how you feel" or "I've had similar concerns myself" can serve to validate a patient's concerns, to open avenues of communication, and to create important symmetries between two persons in a room.

The Physician

Case 3

Mr. V, an impeccably dressed, fastidious 47-year-old single white male, works as a principal in a private high school. On presentation to a university psychiatric clinic, Mr. V describes "anger and frustration" relating to his experiences at work. Many of the "younger teachers" had threatened his "authority" by questioning long-standing rules of order in faculty meetings. Initially, Mr. V had "tried to reason with the miscreants" by explaining that he, as principal, was solely responsible for running meetings. When this failed Mr. V reacted harshly, banning several young faculty members from meetings, while attempting to censor others. These procrustean ways did not go over well at all. Many faculty members signed a petition calling for his ouster. And the school headmaster, in direct response, called for a "more flexible" style of school leadership. On the intake form Mr. V describes feeling "depressed" as a result of these events—"pessimistic," unable to sleep, unsure of how to act at work, constantly worried he would lose his job, and unable to enjoy life.

On the first clinic visit Mr. V is assigned to the care of a PGY-IV resident. As Dr. R, a 28-year-old woman, enters the room, Mr. V voices annoyance. "I will only be seen by a senior physician," he demands. When it is explained that this is not possible, Mr. V becomes increasingly upset, refusing to speak with the resident. Eventually the clinic supervisor accompanies the resident into the examining room to explain the rules of engagement. Begrudgingly, Mr. V describes his symptoms to Dr. R, and is prescribed an SSRI antidepressant. In the subsequent three sessions Mr. V is increasingly late, and spends the majority of the allotted time complaining of a vast array of side effects, including "blurred vision," "agitation," and "headache." Near the conclusion of the third session, Mr. V threatens to discontinue the medication, stating that "these medications don't help me at all." Dr. R then seeks to refer Mr. V to the care of another resident in the clinic.

To complicate matters, in supervision after the third session, Dr. R describes a strong negative reaction to Mr. V. As she explains, the patient had elicited feelings of anger and resentment. She recalls "the principal I always hated," and an uncle who had been exceedingly strict when she was a child. Understandably she experienced the patient's undermining of her authority as overbearing, and as potentially sexist and discriminatory. As a result, Dr. R realizes, she initially sought to reestablish control of the interview. As her anger grew, she refrained from asking open-ended questions that might have established a closer connection with Mr. V—such as "How are you feeling?" Instead, her questions became increasingly concrete—"Do you have allergies to medications?" "Have you experienced nausea?"—eliciting ever-shorter answers. The result in effect limited the amount of time spent with the patient. While this may have been the case, this strategy also led to a breakdown in the exchange of important information. This left Mr. V feeling "angry and misunderstood," and with the feeling of being controlled, thus setting a tone of impersonal interactions and resistance that would continue throughout future sessions.

This brief case description serves to illustrate several levels of difficulty for the clinician attempting to form a therapeutic connection with a patient such as Mr. V. Mr. V demonstrates many of the potential, patient-centered blocks to communication discussed in the previous section. Moreover, the transference in such a case, whereby a young clinician represents a threat to an older principal, presents its own series of complicated issues. And yet the case of Mr. V hints at the ways in which obstacles to the therapeutic collaboration can involve the physician as well. A physician's responses, his or her understanding of the clinical role, or his or her reaction to the patient, can all greatly alter the course of the inter- action. While these responses will be further explored in Chapter 5, they are also important to consider in the context of the therapeutic alliance.

Strategies. It is normal for a physician to experience any number of emotional responses to a patient. Like a patient, a physician enters the clinical encounter with a series of biases and points of view. Moreover, pa- tients with character pathologies are often quite adept at eliciting strong emotional responses from caregivers. These can range from anger, to hos- tility, to arousal. Patients who are depressed, or who are psychotically withdrawn, can elicit feelings ranging from helplessness to overprotect- edness. And understandably, patients who are potentially violent can po- tentiate feelings of fear.

In the case of a medication interaction, however, it is exceedingly im- portant that a physician be able both to reflect upon his or her reactions, and to realize that these reactions open a window into the internal work- ings of the patient. Moreover, he or she must always be mindful of the ways in which medications can become implicated in the patient's ex- pressive system, and specifically in the patient's modes of communication with the clinician. Medications can serve as points of resistance, or as ve- hicles of acting out. Such communication can be made manifest by over- dose or by discontinuation, by forgetting to take one's medications, or by "innocently" and "accidentally" spilling them upon the floor during a fol- low-up exam. This realization on the part of the therapist is important for two reasons. First, it is likely that the impediments the patient enacts in clinical encounters are similar to those constructed in the patient's life. And second, this awareness will lessen the possibility that tensions will be mediated through the prescription of medication.

To address the issue of countertransference, clinicians should con- tinually examine—either internally or in supervision—the specific as- pects of a clinical situation that can lead to a negative response. Questions might include the following: When does the clinician first become aware of feeling uncomfortable or angry? What is the experience at that time? It is a threat to authority? a loss of control? a reminder of an earlier relationship? And, importantly, What response did such emotions elicit? Did they cause defensiveness? a need for containment of emotional re- sponses? anger? In a stable, long-term clinical relationship, such infor- mation can be discussed with patients (Gabbard, 1999). More frequently, however, the awareness of such responses are part of the metadiscourse through which a clinician becomes aware of his or her role. A more complete discussion of this process will follow in subsequent chapters.

The System

Case 4

Ms. P is a 23-year-old graduate student in political science who has been in psychotherapy for the past 2 years. Over the course of this time period she has formed a close working relationship with her therapist, a licensed social worker, whom she sees twice weekly. Throughout her treatment Ms. P has adamantly voiced antipathy to the possibility of psychotropic medications. She had been treated with antidepressants as a child, and remembers the experience to have been intensely painful. However, Ms. P's depressive symptoms have worsened considerably in the preceding months. She has lost her appetite, her ability to sleep through the night, and her enjoyment of life. In spite of her own reservations about psychotropic medications, Ms. P's therapist eventually advises Ms. P to seek psychiatric consultation. It turns out, however, that the psychiatrist with whom the therapist usually works is not covered by Ms. P's insurance. Ms. P then visits a psychiatrist provided by her health plan.

Ms. P arrives 15 minutes late for her evaluation with the psychiatrist. She enters the physician's office and sits down without explanation. In terse, short sentences, she voices a great deal of reservation about "telling my problems to a complete stranger."

It was once believed that the therapeutic alliance was formed in closed dialogue between two parties whose roles were clearly demarcated. A patient spoke, while a clinician listened and interpreted. In time, speaker and listener were able to fuse into a cohesive unit, and in the process, to overcome the resistance that stood in their way. In an age of managed care and medication referrals, however, this notion of dialogue is called into question, if not entirely replaced. Both doctor and patient are forced into continued awareness of third and often fourth parties, or of relationships—and potentially deeper relationships—existing outside of the immediate encounter. This awareness is often acutely realized in a medication consultation, where the terms of engagement between doctor and patient can serve to directly threaten the possibility of a therapeutic bond. The case of

Ms. P speaks to the difficult negotiations that must take place when a patient is referred by a therapist. A patient might feel as if his or her alliance with the therapist is threatened by the possibility of a new clinical encounter. Should the clinician prescribe medications, this new relationship will be ongoing. Such conflicting tensions can greatly effect care. For example, the conflict of psychotherapist and prescribing psychiatrist might cause patients to minimize symptoms, to engage in therapeutic splitting (whereby providers are polarized into categories of "good" and "bad"), or to react in a negative manner toward the psychiatrist.

Strategies. In such cases clinicians are forced to realize that clinical arrangements are not really dialogues. Rather, and ever increasingly, they involve three or four providers, and numerous other interests. Clinicians need to be able to negotiate this algebra. This is accomplished by maintaining an awareness of the other relationships at play, and keeping open avenues of dialogue. Clinicians should continually discuss decisions, progress, and treatment plans with referring therapists. As Imhoff et al. (1998) argue in the article "The Relationship between Psychiatrist and Prescribing Psychotherapist,"

> . . . unless the treating therapist and prescribing psychiatrist have a mutually respectful working relationship, unless they are aware of the ways in which the strength and cohesiveness of their relationship may affect the treatment outcome, and unless they develop a collaboration that sustains the integrity of both the patient-therapist relationship and the patient-prescribor relationship, the prognosis for a successful treatment experience will be significantly compromised. (p. 262)

Attitudes toward Medication

As medications increasingly become cultural symbols, a clinician needs to keep the notion of stereotypes and metaphors at the fore of clinical communication. Many patients have preconceived notions about medication based on what they hear on television or read in magazines.

Case 5

Elise F is a 21-year-old financial analyst who suffers from social phobia. In the opening moments of her initial visit to a psychiatrist, she explains, "I've seen a Prozac advertisement in *Marie Claire* magazine, and realize that I have a chemical imbalance. I believe that I need Prozac to correct this."

In an era when the chemical imbalance is common parlance, and when medications such as Prozac are discussed as the miracle cures to chemical rebalance, psychotropic medications can function as fetishized commodities. Patients may present to psychiatrists specifically requesting brand-name medications, and can experience a sense of rejection if their expectations are not met.

In a climate in which psychotropic medications are construed as commodities, a clinician must at least consider the ways that illnesses such as depression, and medications such as antidepressants, are defined in popular culture as well as in medicine. To be sure, the past decades have seen great advances in understanding the genetic and biological bases of these illnesses. And the DSM-IV provides well-tested criteria for identifying its clinical manifestations. However, the signs and symptoms of depression are also increasingly delineated in popular culture as well. Advertisements, for example, promote depression and its brand-named treatments to the millions of consumers who read popular magazines. Employing bright color graphics and Keith Haring styles, these images mix contemporary fashion with state-of-the-art technique to shape the ways women consumers think about, and indeed talk about, depression. And, since physicians are part of this same culture, and since many of the same advertisements concomitantly appear in professional journals, these advertisements can serve to shape the ways physicians discuss depression as well.

The case of Elise F thus broaches the controversial topic of direct-to-the-consumer advertising of pharmaceuticals, and lets us think briefly about the effect these advertisements might have upon the clinical interaction of doctor and patient. In August 1997, the U.S. Food and Drug Administration significantly relaxed regulations on the site and content of pharmaceutical advertisements. Subsequently, advertisements that had once been directed solely at physicians began to appear in magazines such as *Cosmopolitan, Self,* and *Marie Claire,* and on television, billboards, and radio. As the titles of these magazines suggest, the advertisements have been directed primarily at young women. Women are almost twice as likely as men to be diagnosed with, and treated for, depression. Numerous articles and editorials have accused advertisers of seeking to play upon, and to expand, these imbalances of epidemiology (Zita, 1998). Supporters of pharmaceutical advertisements, meanwhile, contend that these advertisements provide important sources of information.

Strategies. To be sure, the prevalence of information about medications has meant widespread destigmatization, increased awareness, and improved levels of care (Healy, 1997). However, discussions based upon direct requests for products often risk overgeneralization and misunderstanding if not adequately explored. For example, the notion of a "chemical imbalance" might signify widely disparate definitions to different patients. These can range from a patient's desire to "not look too deep" at emotional issues, to a feeling of potentially gendered peer pressure tied into the perception of SSRI antidepressants as technologies of "personal enhancement" (Parens, 1998). Similarly a physician's rush to prescription based upon culturally coded terminology might be made in haste, or might be experienced by a patient as a caregiver's lack of interest.

Simply stated, neither catchphrases such as "chemical imbalance," nor specific requests for brand-name medications, should go unexplored. Rather, a clinician needs to assist each patient to unpack the meaning of such terminology whenever possible (Bersani, 1986).

Elise F's presenting request, for example, might allow for a series of open-ended questions. With what in the advertisement did she identify? What did "chemical imbalance" mean to her? Why did she seek Prozac specifically? What did she expect the results of such treatment to be? Did she feel these to be plausible goals?

The purpose of refusing to take "information" such as stereotypes or cultural slogans at face value is fourfold. First, this line of questioning helps weed out improper requests. Second, by probing the meaning of stereotype and metaphor, a clinician can address the possibility that these rhetorical tropes might be masking deeper symptoms or unexpressed emotions. Third, such questions allow for a discussion of potentially unrealistic expectations, either positive or negative. Given the host of complicated cultural and cross-cultural meanings of medications, only a few of which are present in the case of Elise F, these expectations are important to put on the table at the outset of treatment. And finally, addressing the meaning beneath the oversimplification creates the beginnings of a more thoughtful conversation, thus enhancing what can sometimes feel like a potentially impersonal bond between consumer and physician. Whether or not a medication is ultimately prescribed, a consideration of the symbolic value of medications can be as important to understanding its clinical efficacy as is the awareness of its direct effects (Metzl, 2000).

CONCLUSION

In a harried and ever-more technical world, an understanding of the therapeutic bond between patient and physician might seem a relic of a bygone era. To be sure, relationships, allegiances, and modes of information exchange continually evolve. In the medical system, this evolution has been catalyzed by many of the factors presented above—ranging from the changing beliefs and presuppositions both parties carry into (and then enact within) the examination room, to the often-impersonal alterations in the medical system, to the impact of cultural and cross-cultural perception. Such shifts have in many ways threatened classical notions of alliance formation. However, beneath a veneer of postmodern disconnect, the therapeutic interaction is at its core a relationship between two people, doctor and patient, in a room. Continued attention to, and discussion of, the nuances of their interaction enhance the possibilities of a successful, and indeed a personally meaningful outcome for both parties involved.

CHAPTER THREE

Using the Interview to Establish Collaboration

Case 1

Mr. A, a 21-year-old extremely psychotic man, was admitted to the inpatient unit of a general psychiatric hospital. The therapist sees Mr. A for the first time standing in the hallway of the unit, and goes up to him to introduce himself. He sticks out his hand to greet Mr. A, who stands rigidly with his arms at his sides.

> Dr. A: I would like to talk to you today.
> Mr. A: You are.
> Dr. A: I would like to see you sometime today.
> Mr. A: You are.
> Dr. A: (*Thinks to himself, "What a hostile guy this is, but I'll give it one more try."*) Later on in the afternoon I would like to meet with you in my office on the first floor.
> Mr. A: Sure (*and then slowly walks away*).

Later in the day Dr. A approaches Mr. A, who recognizes him, and together they go off, without difficulty, to Dr. A's office on the first floor.

Case 2

Mr. B, 35-year-old vice president of a small company, was sitting up in bed in the medical emergency room. He had taken an overdose of paroxetine and alprazolam because his wife had just filed divorce papers that day. He appeared to be wide awake when the psychiatrist arrived to interview him, and initially he spoke in a clear, full voice but all he could say was: "I was stupid to try to kill myself. I thought the world would be better off without me."

However, when the psychiatrist began to ask him more questions, his speech became slurred, his voiced softened considerably, and he seemed to drift off into light sleep. After a number of attempts to try to get him to respond to his questions, the psychiatrist remarked:

DR. B: You know, I have a problem with this. My job is to try to decide whether or not you should be in the hospital, and if I cannot understand what you are saying, then I don't know how I am going to make the correct decision.

MR. B: (*interrupting and speaking more clearly*) I don't want to be in the hospital. I just did a stupid thing.

DR. B: I know you think that. You said that before. But I need to be able to sit down and have a conversation with you if I am to make a decision that I think is right. I want to do the right thing, but the right thing may or may not be what you want. But if we could talk together for a while, that is, if you could stay awake, try not to slur your words as much, and speak a little louder, I think we could decide on something that would work for you, and what we decide might even be the right thing.

Mr. B began to talk louder and more clearly, and began to provide elaborated answers to questions. After about 20 minutes of conversation, both he and the psychiatrist agreed that Mr. B didn't have enough support at home at the moment for him to feel safe there. And he had no other place he felt he could go to in lieu of going home. They both agreed that a short stay in the hospital would give Mr. B and the hospital staff a chance to line up support and therapy for him. He was admitted without incident.

There is no one way to interview a patient, either in the initial, follow-up, or subsequent interviews (MacKinnon & Michels, 1971). The main task of any psychiatric interview is to provide a setting for dialogue that can be as open as possible and still obtain specific information. Another important task is to maintain that dialogue while building some semblance of mutual trust between the interviewer and the patient. This trust not only involves trust between the two people, but trust in the process of a patient going to see a psychiatrist. During the interview, both patient and psychiatrist should be feeling each other out. Another task is the maintaining and strengthening of that trust and relationship, so that not only from the outset, but also throughout the course of the treatment, the patient takes on the role of being a partner in the medication-prescribing and maintenance process.

The initial interview is crucial in that it provides an opportunity to establish the context in which the remainder of the treatment, whether medication management or psychotherapy or some combination of both, will be conducted. No matter what eventual type of treatment will be undertaken, the same initial interview should be conducted.

Nonetheless, more and more frequently today the initial interview focuses on deciding on a diagnosis and determining the proper medication for the treatment of a person with that particular diagnosis. Even when one is assigned the role of purely being the medication manager, the importance of the initial interview cannot be underestimated. This interview may be the only opportunity to gather vital information, from the psychiatric, social, medical, and interpersonal spheres, to allow us to make a reasoned and informed diagnosis and decision about medication. In addition it is an opportunity to set the tone for the nature of the interpersonal relationship that will exist throughout the course of the treatment.

The initial interview can be divided into four distinct parts:

1. An open-ended stage where the physician allows the patient to expand upon the chief complaint. During this phase of the interview, questions should be asked primarily to encourage the patient to expand upon and elaborate the circumstances of her current life and how her complaint(s) fit into that life. The goal is to find out something about who the patient is.
2. An assessment of the patient's perception of what it was like to grow up in her family of origin as well as in her current family constellation, as well as a family history of medical and psychiatric disorders.
3. A symptom-based assessment where the psychiatrist probes for the presence or absence of specific psychiatric symptoms that come together into syndromes that are the DSM psychiatric diagnoses. Questions should address previous trials with psychiatric medications and current medications (both psychiatric and nonpsychiatric), and allergies, and ongoing and current medical problems. A formal mental status examination, if necessary, is conducted during this phase.

4. Finally, a presentation and discussion of treatment plan, treatment contract, and medications chosen. Patient input is crucial here.

This chapter will review those stages and will also discuss difficulties in the process and how they might be overcome.

GENERAL PRINCIPLES OF THE INTERVIEW PROCESS

When a patient appears in the emergency room and states that he or she is depressed, too often the interview rapidly turns into a recitation of questions that sounds like a symptom checklist. The goal of the questions is to clarify whether the patient has a major affective disorder or whether or not the patient endorses a sufficient number of criteria for a major depressive episode as set forth in DSM-IV (American Psychiatric Association, 1994). This process might, in essence, insure that the proper diagnosis has been made and lead to appropriate decisions regarding the most efficacious treatment. From our point of view, something major has been omitted from the process. At the end of a thorough diagnostic interview, the interviewer may still know nothing at all about who the patient really is, what makes him tick, or how the current episode fits into who he is and into his life.

In addition, we need to consider the fact that depression, as an example, is not only a diagnostic entity but is also an adjective used to describe a mood state or affect. The patient doesn't think of depression in the clinical psychiatric sense but instead is using a word that helps him describe his mood state. We are suggesting caution in that we should not automatically assume that we know what a patient means when he uses a word that is ambiguous or can have multiple meanings. We need to inquire what the word means to that particular patient. We are reminded of the vaudeville interchange that begins with the question, "How did you arrive at the theater?" (implying a question about career choice and path), and meets the retort, "By bus!"

Thus we recommend a beginning series of questions or prompts that allows, in fact, that encourages, the patient to expand and to develop his story.

Case 3

Dr. C: What is happening that leads to your coming to the emergency room?

Ms. C: I am depressed.

Dr. C: Can you tell me about your depression?

The above interchange will lead to a very different response and thus a very different data set than the following interchange:

Dr. C: What is happening that leads to your coming to the emergency room?

Ms. C: I am depressed.

Dr. C: Do you cry a lot?

You could replace the last line with any symptom-oriented question, "Are you having trouble sleeping?" or "Has your appetite changed?" or "Are you hopeless and helpless?", and find yourself able to tick off the symptoms on a checklist. This response is entirely different than responding with the following question: "Can you tell me about your depression?" While it is essential to find out about sleep, appetite, motivation, sex drive, and so forth, you don't want to start with a series of symptom-based questions, but rather allow the patient to elaborate in his or her own words the psychiatric or psychological dilemma or life problem. This helps us understand what the patient means by depression in his or her life and conveys to the patient that his or her feelings matter. Further, this approach avoids considering the patient merely as an entity that needs to be classified ("Have you seen/felt/palpated/discussed that terribly hard nodular liver on the sixth floor?"). This open approach shows the patient you see him or her as a unique individual with feelings, problems, and an admixture of many things that has led him or her to believe that he or she is in an emotional crisis ("Have you met that young fellow on the sixth floor with liver cancer? Isn't that tragic? He has so much potential. And he is acting so brave about the whole thing, but I know he is really depressed. And the examination of his liver, its hardness and dullness affirms how dire his situation is"). There are a number of key differences in the phrasing that include "seen" versus "met," "liver" versus "young man," as well as the complexity of the patient's feelings and presentations "brave . . . but . . . really depressed."

The Initial Interview

What follows are some principles and processes that we think should take place in the initial interview with any patient in any setting. The interview process suggested is not designed specifically for medication management or for psychotherapy or for some combination of both. It is not meant to be used solely on the inpatient unit or in the Emergency Room or for the initial appointment in an ambulatory setting. Rather, it is an interview that we believe will allow the psychiatrist to obtain basic psychosocial and medical/biological information within the time period of about an hour while appreciating who the patient is, how she thinks, and what matters to her. What is presented may at first sound like an overly ambitious assignment; yet if done correctly, the interview can easily be accomplished in a smooth and empathic way that lays the foundation for a strong doctor-patient relationship. The time and the tactical approach of the interview, perhaps, would need to be modified for people with severe mania or psychosis or an advanced organic brain syndrome, and it certainly would need to be modified if less than 45 minutes to an hour were allotted for the interview.

A comment perhaps is in order regarding the length of time allotted for the initial interview. Many psychiatrists working for managed care companies or in managed care settings state that they are allotted only 15 or 20 minutes per patient. While this may be somewhat adequate for medication follow-up appointments, it seems woefully inadequate for an initial interview, even if another initial interview has been conducted by another person, such as a nonmedical therapist or a primary care physician. First, the type of psychiatric interview we are proposing is not the same as a psychological assessment done by a nonmedical therapist. This type of interview is not something that can be considered complete after conducting only a thorough review of systems accompanied by determining that the patient has a particular score on a screening instrument such as the PRIME-MD (Spitzer et al., 1994) even if that review of systems is embellished with a series of more direct questions about psychiatric symptomatology. Rather, the psychiatric interview we are proposing encompasses an exploration of social (stressors, living situations, social support, socioeconomic status and responsibilities), psychological (cognition, defensive organization, characterological and temperamental elements), and psychiatric (i.e., symptoms and syndromes of psychopathology) aspects of a given individual in both a structured and unstructured format. Similarly, one could then argue that an hour is really insufficient to gather all this information. Nonetheless, we propose that an interview that follows the structure (there is structure even to the "unstructured" parts) and rhythm as discussed below should provide enough basic information for the treating psychiatrist to make an informed decision regarding medications while establishing rapport with the patient. And hopefully, in the process, the psychiatrist can begin to lay the groundwork for a doctor-patient relationship that will help sustain the treatment and enhance compliance. If the organization that one works for does not allow 45 to 60 minutes for an initial interview, the argument needs to be made that sufficient time allotted to an initial interview will lead to better treatment, more rational and more cost-appropriate medication decisions, and a greater overall knowledge of the patient that can help prevent adverse reactions and the medical and legal consequences that can follow such an event.

As we return to our initial dialogue with the patient who says, "I am depressed," we believe the psychiatrist's response should be something like "Tell me about your depression," or "What does it mean to you when you say you are depressed?", or "What is going on with you that leads you to think that you are depressed?" Each of these phrases is put forth in order to accomplish the same end, which is to allow the patient to expand on his description. Perhaps he will immediately list a number of stressors at work or at home, talk about marital difficulties, the death of a parent, a financial setback, a failed relationship, a missed "golden opportunity," a situation that has caused him overwhelming fear, a rejected love, a poor grade on a paper, an argument with a roommate, an inability to eat, sleep, concentrate, or get any enjoyment out of life for no good reason, or one of thousands of other events/topics that each of us could imagine and suggest. But few, unless they are well-practiced psychiatric patients, will say, "Well, I know I'm depressed because I am blue, cry a lot, feel helpless and hopeless, can't get pleasure out of anything, have a phase shift in my sleep, and want to kill myself." Even if a patient replies simply with "Because I want to kill myself," we suggest a reply, "Wanting to kill yourself may come from many different things. Can you tell me what's going on with you that makes you want to kill yourself?" Again, we do not deny that there is much more specific work to do around the statement of wanting to kill himself, such as Is there a plan, Are there weapons available, has he ever tried to kill himself before? But these questions come later. At this stage of the interview, the goal of the interviewer should be to get the patient to elaborate on feelings and to probe where the interviewer thinks there is a vein rich with psychological ore.

Case 4

Mr. D. was a 48-year-old married man who came under his own volition to the emergency room in an extremely intoxicated state. He was given some water, accompanied to the bathroom and allowed to wash up, and told he could wait, if he thought he could do that quietly, until he felt he was able to talk with the psychiatrist. About an hour later, he tearfully approached the clerk and said he was ready to talk.

DR. D: How long have you been drinking?

MR. D: Just tonight.

DR. D: Just tonight?

MR. D: Yes, just tonight. Don't you believe me?

DR. D: Well, you look a mess. What's the story?

MR. D: The story is that my mother died last week. I have a sister who has been in the state mental hospital since she was 22, and I haven't seen her for years. In fact, I don't even know if she is still alive, but I guess my mother or I would have been notified. Anyway, I think I need to call her and tell her our mother died but I am terrified to do that alone. I just started drinking and crying and feeling guilty about ignoring her but also knowing I needed to call her. Listen, I need your help, Doc. Can I call her from here and would you stand by me just in case I freak out or she freaks out?

Our plan, to which Mr. D agreed, was first to allow us to call his wife. We called her, she took him home overnight to become sober and clean up. He came back to the Emergency Room the next day and was assisted in the call to his sister.

As the patient elaborates on these issues, the therapist's posture is twofold. The therapist should listen to everything as the truth, that is, believe that what the patient is relating to us is the truth or at least that everything has the power of truth to the patient. At the same time, the therapist needs to be skeptical of everything the patient tells her. The therapist should be listening for contradictions and inconsistencies, for things that seem impossible to have occurred, and for things that just don't make any sense at all. One listens at this point not with the goal of pointing out the inconsistencies or the hard-to-believe statements, but rather to gain information about a number of different things concerning the patient. We have the opportunity to learn how the patient thinks and sees his world. We gather information that will help us to formulate future questions that might clarify inconsistencies in the patient's narrative while providing us with information on the patient's ability to see himself. We will learn about the complexity of the psychological world in which the patient lives, and with this understanding, we will be able to be more readily empathic with the patient's situation. (In the clinical vignette in case 4, it was reasonably clear from the organization of Mr. D's speech [" . . . but I guess my mother or I would have been notified"] that he was not a chronic user of alcohol.)

We must never forget that patients arrive at their symptomatology honestly, that is, that almost all people try to do their best with their own limited psychological, social, and/or financial resources. As people make choices, they may find themselves on a narrower and narrower path where choices are limited and the path becomes, for the patient, a thin corridor from which there seems little chance to deviate or escape. This is true whether one ascribes psychopathology to biological or developmental sources, or to a combination of both.

Also we are listening for themes in each elaboration. Does the patient always wind up seeing himself as the victim? Does the patient always feel that she is brighter than anyone else in the situations that have been elaborated upon? Does the patient feel that he is never fully appreciated? Does the patient repeatedly blame others for her choices and thus the consequences that befall her? Is the patient frankly paranoid? If a patient repeatedly does not notice his inconsistencies (something we all do probably a lot more regularly than most of us would care to admit), it may say something about the patient's ability to step back and look at himself, or something about the patient's need to impress, or something about the patient's feeling of whether or not you take him seriously.

To listen with skepticism does not mean to not take the patient seriously. On the contrary, to listen while simultaneously believing and being skeptical involves a tremendous amount of concentration and thoughtfulness on our part. We are listening to the patient on many levels. We are listening to the narrative as well as listening for the underlying themes embedded in the narrative. We are listening to whether or not the affect expressed is consonant with the narrative (if any affect at all is being expressed), and we are trying to determine whether all of this makes narrative and emotional sense.

Case 5

Ms. E, a 28-year-old married woman, mother of two young children, had been held hostage by a stranger for no explicable reason. The kidnapping lasted for about 56 hours. During the period of the kidnap, there had been threats with weapons, little food or water, rare opportunities to use the bathroom, and the constant use of handcuffs or ropes to keep her tied up and restrained. Two aspects of the patient's account of this harrowing episode stood out to the therapist. The first aspect was that the patient was very oriented to detail about when, what, and where things happened. The patient would spend an inordinate amount of time wanting to get it "exactly" right. (It would eventually be brought to light in later sessions that she felt that her parents never believed what she said, and she needed to be sure that the therapist believed what she said so she supplied all these actual details to bolster the "truth.") While the patient struggled with the details, the therapist remained quiet and allowed the patient the time to "get it right." The therapist felt that the patient's concentrating on the details allowed her to control as well as to be distracted from the overwhelming emotions attached to this event. This need to account for detail did not neatly fit into the therapist's hourly schedule, and after three sessions, each a week apart, the patient had only gotten through recounting the first day.

The therapist knew he had a large block of time that had unexpectedly become available to him and thus was unscheduled the following week, and he suggested, if the patient thought she wanted to, that they could utilize a 4-hour block of time. She said that that would be OK with her, and so they met. It took her 3½ hours of further detail before she could finally say, "Well, that's what happened." The second aspect was that throughout the entire marathon session as well as during each of the previous three hourly appointments, the patient was essentially affectless as she went over the events in minute detail. Except for some self-denigrating sarcastic remarks and an occasional ironic laugh, all the sessions were devoid of affect. Yet her own descriptions of herself were certainly not of an affectless person. And despite her lack of affect, the therapist experienced the telling of her narrative of the kidnapping as one of the most powerful affective encounters in his life. Her fear, her bravery, her intelligence, her will to live, her quickness and solidity of thought in the face of real danger, her ability to contain her panic, and her eventual release added to the affective power of the narrative. With no affect from her but with a room full of affect, there was a long silent pause after the patient finally said, "Well, that's what happened." Then the therapist began to cry. Someone had to let go of the feelings. The patient probably was willing to release the facts but held back on the affect even though the affect filled the room. Her inability or unwillingness to release the affect became the sudden and surprising release of affect by the therapist.

Thus if a patient is allowed to expand upon what it is that he or she feels, much can be learned. And what is learned is not merely the feelings and "facts" of the patient's life, and not merely how the two fit together. By allowing the patient to expound, we learn a lot about how he or she thinks, how well his or her thoughts are organized, whether there is a smooth flow of thought and speech, whether there are clearly illogical cognitive errors, whether thought is tangential or circumstantial or clearly psychotic, whether thought and speech deteriorate with time, whether the patient is of average or above-average intelligence, and whether the patient is looking at us and relating the story to us or just talking it to anyone who might be sitting and willing to listen. In other words, does the patient acknowledge and relate in any real way to the other person in the room? All these are details of what one might include in parts of the formal description of the Mental Status Exam (MSE), and they can be readily gathered from this type of interview without having to ask a single question directed solely to establishing data for the MSE. Thus we are able to collect very specific data while allowing the patient the privilege of telling us his or her story in an unstructured, smooth narrative that is an essential part of the interview.

The first part of the initial interview should be conducted in this manner. The second part of the interview should be divided into two parts (see Table 3.1). The first part (of the next section of the interview) should focus on family history, within both the family of origin as well as the current family constellation in which the patient is living. When one focuses on family history, one should not initially focus solely on family medical or psychiatric history ("Has anyone else in your family been depressed or alcoholic?") but rather on how the patient perceived his family when he was growing up ("Could you tell me something about what your family was like when you were growing up and what it was like for you to be in that family?"). After gathering some information as to the patient's feelings and memories, then we can transition into the more question-and-answer part of the interview. ("Did anyone else in your family have psychiatric or other emotional problems?"). A few more specific questions about family medical and substance abuse history can then easily lead back to asking about the more specific criteria related to the chief complaint which, in the example we are using, is depression. We call this the second part (of this section) of the interview. At this juncture specific queries as to sleep, appetite, sexual drive, variation of mood, and so forth can be asked. Many other depression criteria have also been assessed during the open narrative part of

TABLE 3.1. The Initial Interview

Process	Goals	Time[a]
An open-ended phase where the physician allows the patient to expand upon the chief complaint.	Find out who the patient is and how the patient thinks.	20–25 minutes
An assessment of the patient's perception of growing up in his or her family of origin; assessment of current family constellation including family history of medical and psychiatric disorders.	Appreciate the patient's childhood experiences and major sources of identification.	5–10 minutes
A symptom-based assessment where probes for presence or absence of specific symptoms are presented. Questions relating to previous trials of psychotropic medications, current medical problems and current medications, and allergies are included here. Formal mental status, if necessary, is performed.	Arrive at a DSM-IV diagnosis.	20 minutes
Discussion of treatment plan, treatment contract, and current medication recommendations is conducted with input from the patient.	Plan treatment and elicit feedback from patient.	10 minutes

[a]Times are merely guidelines, and the session is calculated as being 60 minutes in length.

the interview without having to specifically inquire about them. Had there been thought blocking or psychomotor retardation? Did the patient repeatedly express ideas of helplessness or hopelessness or give examples of those feelings in the stories and associations to the narrative? Certainly affect and mood can be gleaned from the more narrative portion of session. And finally, there are safety issues that need to be explored further, particularly in the area of harm to self and others.

At this point, the psychiatrist can be as specific as he wishes, for if the initial part of the interview has gone well, the patient has some experience of the therapist as an empathic individual interested in her and not only in her disease or if she should or should not be admitted to the hospital. In addition, the psychiatrist has a great deal of information about the patient—the patient's consistency, responsibility, intelligence, ability to cooperate with the psychiatrist and the interview process, ability to keep thoughts organized during the narrative, honesty, reliability, goals, and motivations.

All these inform the psychiatrist and are invaluable tools in evaluating the seriousness of a planned suicide attempt or strong suicidal ideation. For example, a patient who says she wishes to kill herself and yet claims she cannot go into the hospital because she has an exam coming up at the end of the week can be appreciated differently both as a person and as a suicidal patient if there has been an open-ended part of the interview wherein the patient has talked a lot about school pressures and personal and familial expectations of academic performance. On the other hand, if the psychiatrist has no sense of the patient's academic drive or familial academic expectations but simply "knows" that the patient is suicidal, then the decision to admit or not is being made in isolation from rather than in the context of the patient and her life.

In addition, the patient's answers to the more specific criteria-based questions will probably be more precise and elaborated if some relationship has been established before the interviewer begins to probe. Once the patient has evidence that the psychiatrist is a good listener, is empathic, and is interested in him, the patient is more likely to see himself as a participant in the process rather than a specimen to be checked and examined and sorted into "admit or do not admit." Further, if the patient was feeling helpless and hopeless before coming to the interview, the very fact that a real connection has been made to another human being may mollify those affects and make living less hopeless and in turn more bearable.

Bringing the Initial Interview to a Close

As the interview draws toward a close, the psychiatrist presents her ideas about what might be happening to the patient, what medications (if any) might be helpful to the patient, and what "level and structure of containment" the patient might need (Gunderson, 1978). (Level of containment relates to how much structure and safety the patient will require.) After presenting all this information to the patient, the psychiatrist then asks, "And what do you think about what I suggest?" Inviting the patient's input and reaction during the first interview establishes the principle that the treatment will be a mutual affair. Further, when a patient refuses or objects to a given recommendation or plan, the response should be, "Well, what do you think we should do instead?" This response should be said without annoyance or irritation or facetiousness. Rather, it needs to be said honestly, with a genuine interest in what the patient really thinks and what kinds of alternatives, if any, the patient has in mind. In the earlier example of a student who is suicidal but says she cannot be admitted to the hospital because she has an exam at the end of the week, the response might go something like this:

Case 6

"Well, I think then we both have a problem. Now it's obvious that if you need to study for the exam then perhaps you won't really kill yourself. But that doesn't reassure me enough. I am still worried, and I am not sure it's as impossible to study in the hospital as you think. So I need some more reassurance that you will be okay. And I also am concerned about what you would do if you did or felt you did poorly on the exam. Earlier on when you were telling me about the expectations and pressures you feel from your parents, you related a story about how you got really drunk when you thought you did poorly on that history exam last semester, and I began to worry about your doing something even more dangerous if you wind up thinking that you did poorly on the exam coming up. And I think your own expectations of yourself have become as demanding as what you think your parents' expectations are of you. So I do need some more specific plan and more reassurance than what we have at the moment."

In the above statement, a number of phrases or pronouns are used to help move the interview toward the idea that this is a collaborative relationship, a dialogue between two people and not simply a situation where one person declares and the other follows. Some examples of key words or key phrasings were presented in the first chapter. The idea of a dialogue, of a give and take, of an exchange of information around a problem where input is needed from both people is established from the very outset ("And what do you think about what I suggest?"). The patient is given time to respond, to react, to think, to present alternatives. If the patient does not agree with the plan, then again the psychiatrist calls for dialogue ("Well, what do you think we should do instead?"). This question needs to be said in a tone that reflects genuine interest in the patient's alternative idea(s), and we cannot reinforce too strongly that there cannot be anger, hostility, sarcasm, contempt, or defensiveness embedded within the question. While this may at first seem to be an easy task, it becomes much more difficult with patients who have characterological or other personality issues. A patient who is viewed as sarcastic or manipulative or a chronic substance abuser does not always engender the most positively empathic feelings in us, and even with the best intentions, some of our own annoyance, frustration, or rage may find its way into this particular type of question (Gabbard & Wilkinson, 1994). And personality disordered patients seemed primed to be acutely sensitive to any hint of anger, hostility, sarcasm, contempt, or rejection.

The reply the patient gives at this point (to the question, "Well, what do you think we should do instead?") may not be satisfactory. But rather than just saying "no," the psychiatrist introduces herself into the equation and into the problem ("Well, I think then we both have a problem"). The psychiatrist reveals that some of this decision-making process has to do with not only who the patient is but who the psychiatrist is as well. Different clinicians may be able to tolerate different degrees of risk. Any particular clinician–patient pairing will generate its own unique feelings about risk and will engender different degrees of connectedness. It is not that all clinicians should be trained to be uniformly connected to all types of patients, though I am sure that many of us and many of the patients that we encounter would wish for more consistency in the interaction. Since it is impossible to achieve that consistency, we must be willing, even eager, to enter into a dialogue with our patients until each side is somewhat satisfied. This dialogue then involves a certain amount of self-revelation and/or limitation on the psychiatrist's part ("But that doesn't reassure me enough. I am still worried"), at least as far as what she can and cannot tolerate; and it involves compromise on the part of both parties in the dialogue. (Please note this self-revelation does not include family, personal shortcomings, home situation, etc. Rather, as explained below, it reveals that the psychiatrist is not just a totally blank screen who doesn't acknowledge feelings, concerns, or worries or doesn't admit that there are some things that he or she might want or might not be able to tolerate that perhaps other psychiatrists could.) The dialogue may involve acknowledgment of disagreement, but that disagreement can be expressed in a reasonable and respectful way ("I am not sure it's as impossible to study in the hospital as you think"). It can also, again in the same spirit with which one introduces disagreement, involve a sort of confrontation about what will and will not be tolerated.

> "Earlier on when you were telling me about the expectations and pressures you feel from your parents, you related a story about how you got really drunk when you thought you did poorly on that history exam last semester, and I began to worry about your doing something even more dangerous if you wind up thinking that you did poorly on the exam coming up. And I think your own expectations of yourself have become as demanding as what you think your parents' expectations are of you."

In the very last sentence, the psychiatrist says, "I need" ("So I do need some more specific plan and more reassurance"), which in some ways sets a limit while at the same time suggesting to the patient that in any interpersonal interaction, the other person may not always behave as we wish them to or just go along with whatever we might want. Dialogues such as the one presented here also serve as a model for dialogues with other people in other interpersonal situations.

Summary of the Initial Interview

The initial interview is the crucial period where one has the opportunity to establish the context in which the remainder of the treatment, whether purely medication management or psychodynamic therapy or some combination of both, will be conducted. No matter what eventual type of treatment will be conducted, the same initial interview should be conducted. It has four distinct parts, and the following outline is based upon a 60-minute interview, and the order of each part is important in establishing a dialogue before asking more specific questions (see Table 3.1):

1. An open-ended part where the physician allows the patient to expand upon the chief complaint. The form of the questions asked by the psychiatrist during this phase of the interview should be primarily to encourage the patient to expand upon and elaborate

the circumstances of his current life and how his complaint(s) fit into that life. The goal is to find out something about who the patient is. (20–25 minutes)

2. An assessment of the patient's perception of what it was like to grow up in her family of origin as well as in her current family constellation. At the end of this part of the interview, the psychiatrist should also ask specific questions to determine a family history of specific medical and psychiatric problems. (5–10 minutes)

3. A symptom-based assessment where the psychiatrist probes for the presence or absence of specific psychiatric symptoms that come together into syndromes that are the DSM psychiatric diagnoses, including previous trials with psychiatric medications and current medications (both psychiatric and nonpsychiatric), and allergies and ongoing and current medical problems. (20 minutes)

4. Presentation and discussion of treatment plan, treatment contract, and medications chosen. Patient input is crucial here. (10 minutes)

MAINTAINING AND STRENGTHENING TRUST IN ALL PHYSICIAN-PATIENT INTERACTIONS

As we have pointed out, all our verbal exchanges with the patient need to be carefully thought out. This premise holds true no matter what particular school of psychotherapy we ascribe to. In fact, this premise should hold true for any patient-physician interaction, whether that physician is a psychiatrist, a primary care physician, or an orthopedic surgeon. What we say has an enormous impact upon our patients; even more of an impact than we would wish for in many circumstances. Such interchanges should always be directed toward (1) reinforcing the idea that what we see is really only our portion of what needs to be a conversation or a dialogue and (2) appreciating that the physician's conduct within the dialogue should be a model for the patient in his or her other interpersonal interactions. We may need to occasionally remind ourselves that what we discuss with our patients is not insignificant. It involves illness, long-term functioning, safety, acceptance, self-esteem, and mutual respect. In fields other than psychiatry it may involve the most intimate details of body parts and functioning and matters of life and death and shame and stigma. But

TABLE 3.2. Interviewing and the Interpersonal Relationship

1. The interview provides a setting for the dialogue that promotes the establishment of the interpersonal relationship.
2. Once the dialogue is established, it must be maintained while building a sense of trust between the interviewer and the patient.
3. Trust is established not only between the two people but in the interview process as well.
4. After trust and the relationship is established, they must be maintained and strengthened so that a true collaborative process evolves between patient and physician.

each conversation that we have with our patients provides a genuine opportunity to further mutual respect, admiration, and trust (see Table 3.2).

Case 6

One of us had been an inpatient psychiatric attending for more than 20 years. It was not uncommon for a patient to be admitted 7 or even 10 years after the previous admission. When the attending and the patient would meet again after so many years, it was also not uncommon for the patient to say, "Doc, I remember something you told me 7 years ago. I have never forgotten it." (The attending hoped, each time that such an exchange took place, that what he had said and/or what the patient remembered he had said was at least decent and hopefully even useful in some small but not insignificant way.)

As mutual trust and respect evolves and hopefully strengthens in the course of the treatment, then the patient becomes a true partner in the medication management process. As stated in an earlier chapter, the goal is not to convince the patient to take a medication that she or he dislikes or cannot tolerate. Rather the goal is mutually to move toward a medication regimen where the cost/benefit ratio for the patient is positive, that is, where the therapeutic benefit clearly outweighs the side-effect profile. This cost/benefit ratio will be different for different patients in that (1) each patient is unique and will react in an individual manner to any medication, and (2) some people are more tolerant than other people of side effects. And further, a particular side effect may be more disruptive to one patient than to another. Certainly the fine intention tremor that often is found with lithium is more disruptive to a calligrapher than to a stock clerk; the loss of sexual desire sometimes found with the selective serotonin reuptake inhibitors can be more troublesome to a young man or woman recently married or wishing to enter into some form of intimate sexual relationship than it may be to a 70-year-old widow (though this is used as an example, and we clearly acknowledge the role and the importance of sex and sexual feelings in elderly people).

The point to be made here is that unless we know about the patient, about their social relationships, their employment, their hobbies, their feelings of acknowledging or not acknowledging the use of psychiatric medications, their previous experience of taking both psychiatric and nonpsychiatric medications, their current and past sexual and interpersonal relationships, their fears of being discovered as a psychiatric patient, and myriad other important and relevant issues to the patient, then we cannot with any wisdom prescribe the correct medication for a given patient. We may certainly prescribe the correct medication for a given disease state, but that is very different from prescribing the best medication for a particular patient with a particular disease state. Often a psychiatrist is asked, "What is your favorite antidepressant?", or "What antidepressant do you use most frequently?" There is no correct answer to those questions. There are many antidepressants, antipsychotics, and many mood stabilizers. We should not have favorites among them; rather we should prescribe a specific medication only after we have searched and discovered what is specific/unique about this particular patient, and which medication within a particular class of medications, given the medication's particular side-effect profile, is more appropriate for this particular patient.

CONCLUSION

It is time to return to the initial two clinical example cases presented at the beginning of this chapter but not yet elaborated upon. In Case 1, the example of the very psychotic man, Mr. A, the psychiatrist's first impression was that the patient was being hostile and was attempting to avoid him. The patient seemed to parry each overture the psychiatrist made. The psychiatrist could simply have given up on the task and let the patient be until he had begun to behave differently. But, in truth, the patient was very psychotic and extremely paranoid, and perhaps the patient was understanding each phrase in its most concrete and literal way. If that was so, then in the initial contact in the hallway, the psychiatrist was in actuality "talking" with him and "seeing" him. In fact when the psychiatrist became more specific about future plans ("Later on in the afternoon I would like to meet with you in my office on the first floor"), the patient was very clear that that would be alright with him. The psychiatrist wanted to open up a dialogue, but he needed to find the right combination of words to convey that to the patient. No true dialogue could be established until the psychiatrist realized that the patient was taking and understanding everything in its most literal and concrete way. Fortunately, the psychiatrist was able to chance upon the right combination of words that the patient could filter through his concrete thinking and hear, acknowledge, and respond to him. (It may be worth noting at this juncture, that it was very difficult to establish a true dialogue with this patient over a 15-month course of treatment. The patient remained extremely concrete in all his thinking. When the psychiatrist felt that he and the patient were finally feeling comfortable with each other, the patient would become more paranoid and refuse to see the psychiatrist for a period of time. Yet despite these difficulties, when the patient felt that he was in a real crisis, the psychiatrist was the only person he would speak to. The psychiatrist had a hard time appreciating that he and the patient had a real relationship, probably because of the severity and chronicity of the patient's psychosis.)

In Case 2, the psychiatrist called on what was presumed to be Mr. B's strength to try to put forth what his cooperation or lack of cooperation could lead to. There was information available on the record in the medical emergency room that this man had no prior history of psychiatric illness, and so the psychiatrist made an appeal to his ego. It was as if he was able to talk through the current crisis to the healthy, functioning part of the patient and say, "I know you are miserable, and I hear that. But we need to work together if we are to solve this crisis." While not said in exactly those words, his statement, "But I need to be able to sit down and have a conversation with you if I am to make a decision that I think is right," accomplished the same thing and did it without recrimination. The psychiatrist had an option to simply say to himself that "he is too uncooperative and ill to not be in the hospital, and whether he agrees or not, he is going to be admitted." Surely, things could have gone in that direction, but the patient would have felt resentment and experienced himself as being controlled and demeaned. If this had occurred, then the level of cooperation in the admission process and during the subsequent hospitalization might have been less than optimal. The psychiatrist asked the patient to work with him, to try to talk with him, so that together, through a dialogue, they could arrive at a reasonable plan. This did not take 5 minutes. It took at least 20 minutes, and during that period, not a lot of time was spent on symptoms other than hopelessness and helplessness. Social supports were explored; his deteriorating relationship with his wife was explored. And it was concluded that the man was so overwhelmed that a time-out or respite would let him recover some of his ego and hopefully would lead to his being able to function and make decisions in a more appropriate manner.

We believe, then, that the first task of any interview with any patient is to open some sort of dialogue. Dialogue occurs more readily when the patient feels listened to and where the patient's opinions are respected and options are considered. This cannot be achieved by simply responding to the patient's complaints with a recitation of a symptom checklist. Rather, before we enter into a checklist or symptom review, we need to be passionate about trying to discover in all our patients both who they are and what ails them above and beyond the specific diagnosis. Not only will such a tactic provide us with a broader understanding and appreciation of the patient, it will also provide us with information that will allow us, together with input and reactions from the patient, to make a reasoned choice among the array of medications available.

The patient needs to be reminded constantly that she or he is a part of the treatment team. This is not done by reiterating that phrase to the patient. Rather, it is accomplished by using every opportunity, even crises, to explore what it is the patient is really feeling, what his or her opinion of the crisis is, and how we can work together to get through the crisis even if we can't solve it. Perhaps if we listened more, we would experience fewer demands from our patients to change medications at the first hint of a crisis and at the first emergence of a side effect.

Thus the posture of dialogue and hunger for patient input must be maintained at each and every contact.

CHAPTER FOUR

Enhancing Adherence in the Pharmacotherapy Treatment Relationship

James M. Ellison, MD, MPH

While listening to the final lecture of a recent continuing medical education program, I found myself plagued by the pounding headache that develops when I exceed my capacity to absorb new information. The attendee seated next to me observed as I touched my head, winced, and glanced longingly toward the exit. Displaying his professional expertise in inference, he asked me if anything were the matter. After I mentioned my headache, he reached into his pocket, pulled out two generic-appearing white tablets, and offered them to me sympathetically. "I use these Excedrins when I get a headache," he assured me, "and they work well." My head really hurt, Excedrins were an appropriate recommendation, the convenience of his offer was hard to resist, and he seemed to be a trustworthy professional. I thanked him for the tablets and downed them gratefully. As the lecture went on, however, my thoughts shifted to nagging doubts about how trustingly, in hopes of feeling better, I had taken unmarked pills from a person whom I had not previously known. I began to muse on the factors that come into play every time medications are offered or prescriptions are written, and I was jarred from that pleasant reverie only by the applause that signaled the end of the lecture.

With some pleasure I also noted that my headache was gone and I thanked my now-trusted colleague for his help.

Among the tools at our disposal in the treatment of mental illness, pharmacotherapy is a remarkably powerful intervention. Medications have come to be essential ingredients in the treatment programs for psychotic and bipolar disorders. In the treatment of other mood disorders, medications are now used much earlier in the course of these diseases and for much milder forms of the disease when compared to 10 to 15 years ago. Not uncommonly, these pharmacologic treatments are unaccompanied by formal psychotherapy. Medications play similarly important roles in the treatment of anxiety disorders, personality disorders, and a host of other syndromes and symptomatic states.

Huge amounts of money are spent in the development of new medications that are increasingly more specific and show greater effectiveness with fewer side effects. A wide variety of drugs are available, giving today's prescribing clinicians an exceptional range of agents among which to choose. Taken appropriately, these medications can exert impressively beneficial effects, yet we prescribing clinicians continue to struggle with the most basic of problems: how to get our patients to take the pills that we think they need in the way we think they should. As efficacious as the medications are in research reports and clinical studies, they cannot be effective without moving from the prescription vial to the patient's body. As the introductory vignette attests, the relationship between the prescriber and the patient has a lot to do with whether the patient complies with the taking of the medication.

Despite evidence that taking medications according to appropriate guidelines can significantly reduce morbidity (see, e.g., Melfi et al., 1998), up to half of our patients do not follow our instructions in their use (Butler et al., 1996; Blackwell, 1976; Chen, 1991). Some patients discontinue their pills altogether after a dose or two, others skip their pills on a "good" day, and some attempt to improve an especially bad day by doubling the prescribed dose. Much of this behavior takes place beyond our clinical awareness, or it is revealed (if ever revealed at all), only as we earn the patient's confidence and press for honest and detailed information.

Until recently, the patient's willingness to follow our advice in matters of treatment was universally referred to as "compliance." Compliance is a term that has various meanings, some of which reflect outmoded models of a therapeutic relationship. Webster's definition of *compliance,* for example, includes "friendly or happy agreement" but also "the act or action of yielding to pressure, demand, or coercion . . . often in a servile or spineless fashion . . . conformity in fulfilling formal or official requirements . . . cooperation promoted by official or legal authority or conforming to official or legal norms" (Gove, 1986, p. 465). By contrast, the term *adherence*, defined as "the act of . . . steady or faithful attachment (as to a party, principle, or cause) . . . continued observance" (p. 26), suggests no such hierarchy. Because I intend to emphasize, among other points, how a collaborative and nonhierarchical treatment relationship can help a patient to use medications appropriately, I will use the term *adherence* rather than *compliance* for the remainder of this chapter. I will discuss the factors that I consider most important in promoting adherence and diminishing nonadherence: the patient's level of distress, medication effects, treatment accessibility, and the therapeutic relationship. I will illustrate my ideas on these matters with some clinical vignettes, assembled from patients' histories with details altered in such a way as to protect confidentiality.

LEVEL OF DISTRESS

One of the main reasons for a patient to stop taking medication, understandably enough, is the absence of distress. Why be exposed to potential side effects if you feel fine or reasonably fine in the first place? Without the motivation provided by distress, the use of medication may seem pointless. Unlike silent medical disorders such as hypertension, which is able to develop dangerously without causing subjective distress, the purview of mental health is restricted for the most part to disorders that cause distress either to the patient or others in his support system. Two nonadherence scenarios commonly seen in mental health settings, therefore, are (1) the initially motivated patient who at first acknowledges distress but experiences relief prior to starting the medication, or (2) the patient in distress who does not acknowledge the presence of distress or, if distress is acknowledged, who assigns the distress to an external stressor rather than to an internal psychological state.

Some patients, occasionally to our amazement, improve dramatically while awaiting an initial appointment. The patient who was distressed enough to schedule an evaluation may spontaneously feel better with the passage of a little time or as a result of self-esteem boosted by having taken active steps to obtain help. This happens even more frequently when a delay of several weeks precedes the appointment and this improvement while waiting probably accounts for some of the "no-shows"; that is, the no-show is an indication of the patient's sense that an appointment is no longer needed.

Many psychiatric conditions flare transiently even if recurrently. Between attacks, the patient with panic disorder may prefer not to dwell on his or her difficulties. The patient with an atypical depression or borderline personality disorder may experience a few days of a despair so agonizing that an evaluation appointment is scheduled (and perhaps to the patient's dismay, not scheduled soon enough) but then missed when the patient feels better. The patient whose social phobia or post-traumatic stress disorder is relatively quiescent until provoked by situational factors may experience considerable relief once the stressors subside or are avoided. In each of these disorders, there is unfortunately a likelihood of later symptom recurrence that is amplified without appropriate treatment.

Some patients experience symptoms so severe as to disable their willingness or sometimes even their capacity to take a prescribed medication as directed. In schizophrenic or bipolar patients, for example, adherence problems can at times be traced to the presence of lack of insight, denial of illness, grandiosity, or paranoid delusions (Chen, 1991). Disorganization may be so severe as to preclude engagement in treatment altogether. The severely depressed patient may so pervasively lack energy and motivation that participation in treatment of any kind is simply too difficult to engage in. The anxious patient may fear the effects and side effects of medication so greatly as to avoid taking the prescribed pills altogether or to devise means of reducing potential harmful effects such as secretly taking a smaller dose of the medication than prescribed. Patients with some Axis II disorders may be prone to a type of denial that is associated with the projection or externalization of their difficulties onto those around them but falls short of outright paranoia. At other times, as in the following vignette, the projection may be a manifestation of partially hidden and barely controlled psychotic thinking.

Case 1

Martha A, a 38-year-old former teacher now staying at home to care for her two toddlers, was referred by her individual psychotherapist.

Were the patient's complaints about her marital relationship distorted, the psychotherapist wondered, and might they represent delusions? The pharmacotherapist who assessed Ms. A for medication noted symptoms of major depression and concurred with the fluoxetine already prescribed by her primary care physician. Though prepared to find paranoid ideation about the patient's husband, he found himself impressed at the patient's ability to tell a logical and credible story of a marriage troubled by gradually escalating minor acts of inconsiderateness and hostility. Uncertain at the end of the evaluation session and forbidden the opportunity to gather further information from family members whom she perceived as unsupportive, the pharmacotherapist recommended that projective psychological testing be obtained, reasoning that this might reveal a thought disorder that the patient was adept at concealing. Before the testing appointment could take place, however, Ms. A stopped her medication, fired her individual psychotherapist, took a serious overdose and was brought to the hospital in a floridly delusional state.

Comorbid substance abuse, documented to be a major source of medication nonadherence among schizophrenic patients (Owen et al., 1996), in my experience also obstructs adherence among patients from all other diagnostic groups. Patients told by a well-meaning pharmacist to avoid alcohol altogether while taking a particular medication may, on reflection, choose to avoid the medication and its prescriber instead. Many patients conceal or underreport their use of alcohol, which must be questioned specifically and also investigated repeatedly when there is evidence suggesting concern. Excessive use of alcohol, in addition to interacting pharmacodynamically and pharmacokinetically with prescribed medications, can impair a patient's capacity to adhere to a medication schedule. The importance of obtaining information from collateral informants for accurate assessment of both alcohol use and medication adherence must be emphasized, though the patient who needs to deny his alcohol usage may object when you request consent to contact people who can provide additional information.

Perhaps the symptoms most amenable to target for pharmacotherapy are those that are both ego-dystonic enough to be distressing and yet not severe enough to disable the patient's ability to cooperate in treatment. Some moderate depressions, panic attacks, or new-onset psychotic illnesses are often gratifying to treat for this reason. The patient recognizes the symptoms, wishes them gone, and is willing to take steps to bring about relief. Yet even in these patients, other factors may interfere with the process of taking medication as prescribed.

Based on these considerations, it is clear that treatment adherence can be enhanced by careful diagnostic assessment and case formulation preceding a decision to prescribe. Particular effort can be directed toward identifying target symptoms of sufficient severity to warrant pharmacotherapy, with special attention to the symptoms that the patient experiences as most distressing. Comorbid diagnoses, such as substance abuse or a personality disorder accompanying an anxiety or mood disorder, must be recognized and included in treatment planning. The presence of psychosis and its effects on insight demand the clinician's recognition and appropriate consideration. When denial of illness or externalization of the source of distress are of too great a magnitude to allow voluntary engagement and participation in treatment, a decision must be made as to further treatment efforts. Some patients must be considered to be at least temporarily inappropriate candidates for pharmacotherapy, despite considerably impaired functioning, if they lack sufficient distress or motivation and possess sufficient competence to refuse treatment. For others, a supportive psychotherapeutic relationship can over time provide a context for the development of insight, trust, and a willingness to explore the effects of medications. Finally, it is necessary to take control in some cases and obtain consent for treatment from an appropriately appointed guardian when ability to recognize symptoms and assess the consequences of their presence and the need for their treatment is so limited as to indicate incompetence.

MEDICATION EFFECTS

Every medication has effects that are desirable and effects that are undesirable. The desirable effects, for any specific patient, are considered therapeutic. Effects that are not desired by that patient, even though another might find them helpful, are considered "side effects." The balance between these therapeutic and side effects is an important determinant in adherence. The ability of the clinician to convince the patient to wait out side effects until the full therapeutic effect can be obtained may be an important element in the eventual outcome of the therapeutic/side effect balance.

In one study that polled both patients and their prescribing physicians, side effects were identified by both groups as the most significant contributor to nonadherence (Warner et al., 1994). Discussion of side effects is one of the important elements of the informed consent discussion that precedes elective prescribing. Often, in my experience, a patient will refuse even to begin treatment with a potentially helpful medication merely as a result of hearing about the possibility of certain feared potential consequences of treatment. While risk management advisers suggest the importance of discussing both infrequent life-threatening side effects and more common though benign side effects, my experience is that patients give much more weight to information about the side effects that may impact on the aspects they feel most relevant to quality of life. The possibility of weight gain, impairment of sexual function, fatigue, or insomnia often instill more alarm than discussion of seizures, arrhythmias, and even sudden cardiac death. In the treatment of bipolar patients on lithium maintenance, for example, Gitlin and colleagues (1989) have documented that weight gain and cognitive symptoms are particularly important sources of nonadherence. Clinicians can enhance adherence that would be undermined by side effects in several ways, discussed in the following subsections.

Side Effects Tolerance

Adherence can be aided by choosing a medication with a side-effect profile likely to be tolerable for the specific patient. Depending upon a patient's individualized concerns, one medication may be more likely to be acceptable than another, even though both are regarded as safe and as effective in treating a specific diagnosis. As a general principle, there are now significantly different choices to be made with respect to side-effect profile among each therapeutic class of medications. The side-effect profile of the SSRI antidepressants, for example, may be more acceptable to many patients than that of the older tricyclic antidepressants. One study found greater adherence with SSRIs than tricyclics, especially when the prescribing clinician was not a psychiatrist (Fairman et al., 1998). Among mood regulators, too, there may be significant differences in tolerability. The side-effect profile of divalproex has been claimed to be more acceptable than that of lithium (Weiss et al., 1998) and many clinicians suggest even greater tolerability for some of the more recently marketed anticonvulsant mood regulators such as gabapentin or lamotrigine. Among neuroleptics, the possibility of avoiding the unpleasant and debilitating consequences of extrapyramidal side effects associated with typical agents encourages clinicians to use the newer, atypical agents.

In a more individualized sense, too, the choice of medications should take into account a particular patient's needs. A medication known to be appetite-enhancing may be welcomed by the cachectic patient with a reduced appetite; another, anxious about gaining weight, will refuse the medication on the basis of this side effect. The medication that one patient prefers because it helps him sleep is rejected by another as too sedating. The medication one patient ultimately rejects as too libido-reducing is appreciated and preferred by another who is eager to achieve better control over uncomfortably intense sexual desires.

Case 2

Walter B, a 67-year-old professor with major depression, diabetes, and peripheral arteriosclerotic vascular disease, was treated with paroxetine. As his mood and neurovegetative symptoms improved, he became increasingly aware of difficulty in sexual function apparently associated with that medication. On his own initiative after 3 months of treatment, he stopped his antidepressant abruptly, a decision that led to unpleasant discontinuation symptoms. When he called his psychiatrist to complain of dizziness and nausea, the intolerable sexual dysfunction and reasons for antidepressant discontinuation were discussed. This side effect was improved by the switch to a different antidepressant.

Of course, in order to appreciate which side effects may be more disturbing to any particular patient, the clinician must get to know the patient and the patient's issues prior to prescribing a particular medication.

Side Effects Education

Educating a patient about side effects prior to treatment will allow patient and prescribing clinician to anticipate which side effects may occur and how they might be managed. This education is also an important component of the informed consent process that precedes prescribing for competent patients.[1] Clinicians need to remain aware that patients are likely to receive additional information about their medications from sources

---

[1] For patients adjudicated incompetent, education is still provided but the focus is on making certain this information is offered to the court-appointed individual who will assist in decisions regarding pharmacotherapy.

outside of the pharmacotherapy relationship. Several years ago, Warner and colleagues (1994) reported their finding that patients were more likely to have obtained information through self-help groups or from the *Physicians' Desk Reference* (PDR) than psychiatrists realized. In more recent years, with dramatically increased availability of information via the Internet, it is not unusual for the patient to educate the clinician about a new medication or new use of an old indication. The patient who has taken initiative and gathered information may need extra discussion in order to understand which parts of the information are applicable to his or her treatment. Furthermore, the pharmacist who fills the prescription may voice a concern when the patient is on a medication regimen that is in any way unusual (for example, a dosage exceeding recommended maximum or the use of combinations of medications unfamiliar to the pharmacist). When I hear directly from the pharmacist or indirectly through the patient about such concerns, I like to make sure that the pharmacist, too, becomes educated about the medication regimen. On occasion, mailing the pharmacist an article will broaden her awareness of your treatment approach and enlist her support in your patient's treatment.

Whatever the source of the information, relevance and clarity are crucial.

- The patient should be able to understand at least the names of the medication (brand and generic),
- the rationale for its use,
- how to tell if it is working, what to do if it appears not to be working,
- when and how to take it, what to do if a dose is missed,
- how long the treatment is expected to continue,
- the side effects that the patient would be likely to want to know about (and any serious ones, even if they are very infrequent), possible effects on driving or work, and known interactions with alcohol and other drugs (Anonymous, 1981).

Time spent providing clear patient education is one of the factors correlated with greater patient satisfaction as measured after an initial psychiatric visit (Eisenthal et al., 1983). It is often helpful to supplement the educational discussion with written materials and on occasion to send copies of these materials to the patient's psychotherapist. Such educational information about the medication can be presented in such a way as to invite dialogue, increasing the patient's understanding and engagement in treatment.

The art of enhancing patient adherence to treatment while still providing appropriate patient education requires not only appropriate content but also appropriate style in presentation of information. Ward (1991) noted the limitations of a patient education approach that relies solely on explanation without taking into account patients' individual personality styles. He advocates, for example, providing more global information to the histrionic patient, more detailed information to the compulsive patient. He suggests you should emphasize to a recovering substance abuser the differences between substance abuse and pharmacotherapy. He advocates talking to the patient interested in "alternative treatments" about the fact that even "natural" medications are still drugs. In addition, this patient might not understand that the neurotransmitters affected by prescribed medications are "natural" and the goal is to restore their normal functioning rather than to create a mental state of inappropriately elevated mood or tranquilized calm.

Case 3

Arthur C, a 38-year-old accountant, sought pharmacotherapy for his major depressive disorder outside of his HMO facility and expressed a willingness to pay out of pocket for appointments because he was so disappointed with the limited information his clinician had given him about regarding his diagnosis and treatment. He had been prescribed bupropion SR and had many questions about the drug's mechanism of action, the alternative choices' relative advantages and disadvantages, the proposed duration of treatment, the possible side effects, and what alternative plans would be implemented if treatment failed to proceed as expected. In actuality, the HMO clinician had chosen an appropriate antidepressant and the patient was responding well with minimal side effects. Following an initial session for history gathering and detailed patient education, supplemented by suggestions as to where further information might be found, the patient made no extraordinary demands on the psychiatrist's time for further information.

In contrast, Angela D was a 41-year-old hair stylist who began her session with a warning not to tell her too much about the medication she was to be prescribed, buspirone for her generalized anxiety disorder. "I want something that works, but I'll get every side effect you warn me about." After reassurance about the medication's generally safe track record and brief mention of the most serious, though rare, potential adverse reactions, the patient felt sufficiently informed and took the medication with good results.

Monitoring Side Effects

Continued monitoring of side effects throughout treatment can enhance adherence. It is obviously not sufficient to educate about side effects only at the beginning of a treatment. Rather, as suggested above, the initial discussion about side effects begins an ongoing interactive process of communication about the wanted and unwanted effects of the medication. Retention of the information initially offered may be limited, and thus further discussions simply to impart basic information may be required. New side effects may emerge, some of which may not have been anticipated during the initial discussion. Experiences initially overlooked or tolerated may come in time to be recognized by the patient as real or potential side effects of the medication, and this could potentially undermine treatment adherence. Finally, laboratory assessment consistent with standard practice can help not only to assure the safety of ongoing treatment but also to identify potential hazards (such as the upward creep of TSH that may precede overt symptoms of hypothyroidism in a lithium-treated patient) even before they become matters of clinical concern.

Ultimately, a medication's acceptability requires effective therapeutic actions. Although clinicians recognize that side effects can interfere with patients' willingness to accept or continue taking a medication, data gathered from one group of patients suggested a willingness to endure side effects when they are associated with a medication that is therapeutically effective (Warner et al., 1994). As clinicians, we may occasionally be faced with the unusual task of persuading a patient to discontinue one effective medication in hopes of finding another with more tolerable side effects. This is illustrated in the following vignette:

Case 4

Elwood E, a 42-year-old man long troubled by depression and anxiety, was waiting outside my office door with a pleased expression on his face for the follow-up appointment two weeks after beginning a trial of phenelzine. It seemed odd, however, that he was crouched on hands and knees. As I approached him, he said with some animation,

"This new medication is great! My mood is finally better and my anxiety is gone." I invited him into my office and as he started to crawl across the threshold I asked if he'd prefer to stand. "Sorry," he said, "but I get too dizzy whenever I stand up." For him, dizziness was a small price to pay for the relief of his psychiatric symptoms, though we were soon able to find a way for him to combat the dizziness as well.

When a medication's desirable effects are accompanied by unpleasant or potentially harmful adverse effects, it is often possible to preserve the use of the medication while finding ways to eliminate or alleviate the adverse effects. On other occasions, with the patient's collaboration, a replacement medication may need to be identified in order to achieve a safe and tolerable treatment regimen.

TREATMENT ACCESSIBILITY

Among the barriers to treatment adherence identified by Warner and colleagues (1994), the lack of a supportive life routine was cited by patients as a key factor. Interestingly, 40% of the patients but only 3% of the psychiatrists considered this to be among the top three contributors to nonadherence. This finding suggests that clinicians must be more attentive to the stability of the patient's social and occupational life, since they impact powerfully on treatment adherence.

Case 5

Jennifer F, a 52-year-old woman diagnosed with bipolar mood disorder, borderline personality disorder, and alcohol dependence in remission, lived a life of emotional lability, financial strain, and unpredictable relationships even despite her continued sobriety and the relative stability her medications had conferred on her. In the midst of several disruptive life events and interpersonal stresses including her psychotherapist's vacation, she skipped her appointment with her pharmacotherapist and retreated to the isolation of her room. When the clinician called to check on her, Ms. F angrily asserted that she had flushed all her pills down the toilet. "I was fine before I took them, maybe they're making me sick. I just need to keep busy and not dwell on my feelings."

A treatment plan that supports adherence must take into account the patient's daily routine. The clinician should seek to understand factors in the patient's life that encourage participation in treatment as well as those that make following a regular medication schedule difficult. Psychotherapy, offered collaboratively with the pharmacotherapy by the same or a different clinician, may provide a place to address sources of instability in the patient's life. Finding ways to strengthen a patient's support system, encouraging involvement in community activities and/or peer-support groups, and offering advice regarding services to help the patient with residential, financial, or vocational concerns all can help to increase the stability of the patient's routine.

Patients whose lives are chaotic and unpredictable or who are homeless may not be able to administer a medication daily, let alone three times daily. In addition to the complexity of the medication regimen (Blackwell, 1976), a host of other issues affect the accessibility of treatment and therefore the likelihood of adherence. Finding a prescribing clinician these days, for example, may be a challenge for the patient whose managed care insurance credentials only a limited panel of clinicians or designates only a limited set of facilities as reimbursable sites for treatment. Initially, while in the throes of great distress, a patient may be willing to accept an inconvenient drive in order to obtain services that must be delivered in a designated facility. As time passes, however, and the patient's attention returns elsewhere, the time required to get to an inconveniently located prescribing clinician may become an important contributor to nonadherence. The same may be said of scheduling times for a visit. Patients employed during standard business hours may be dismayed to learn that the prescribing clinician works during those same hours and may not be available for weekend or evening appointments. Seeking efficiency and perhaps responding to pressure from an employer, the patient may attempt to increase the convenience of treatment by seeking to schedule appointments further and further apart, to hold sessions by phone, or even to use Internet teleconferencing.

Case 6

Harriet G, a 63-year-old woman with generalized anxiety and major depression, sought treatment at the academic teaching hospital. She was motivated, partly by fear of mistreatment elsewhere, to locate the expert who would provide flawless treatment. For such expertise, she was willing to drive an hour in each direction and pay out of pocket for a clinician not covered by her insurance. The combination of paroxetine and buspirone reduced her symptoms. Treatment suffered, however, as a result of her gradually increasing reluctance to attend sessions that were expensive and inconvenient. Instead, she began to manipulate her medication doses on her own, keeping her clinician apprized of her medication changes by telephone. The result, not unexpectedly, was a growing sense of alienation from treatment as the doctor-patient relationship became more tenuous, a series of irrational changes in her medication doses, and a recurrence of symptoms.

In general, patients should be discouraged from beginning a treatment that is likely to become burdensome as a result of inconvenience. Continued attendance at sessions and adherence to a medication program is most likely when the location and scheduling of the treatment are convenient and practical.

Discontinuity of care, an increasingly frequent occurrence in the current healthcare environment, can play havoc with adherence to a treatment plan. It is more common these days for clinicians to cycle through a series of jobs rather than to pursue a lengthy career in one location. With each transition, a group of patients is subjected to the stress of meeting a new clinician. The new clinician, assuming responsibility for many patients in various stages of treatment, may fail to know each patient well enough to make wise, and not merely correct, medication decisions. Similarly, patients cycle rapidly in and out of clinicians' practices as their employers change insurers. The result, these days, is a decrease in the likelihood of a long-term association between patient and clinician. Needless to say, adherence to treatment can be adversely affected in a variety of ways. Clinicians unfamiliar with the patient's complete catalogue of current and past medications may not fully understand the reasons for the regimen of medications prescribed by a prior treating clinician. Further, a clinician-patient association that reflects such random pairing of unpredictable duration promotes premature discontinuation of medication and office visits or inappropriate failure to discontinue a medication no longer required.

The expense of medications is widely believed by clinicians to contribute to nonadherence. Certainly the cost of medications is prohibitive to some patients, especially those who live on a limited and fixed income but must purchase new medications that are not available in a generic form. The survey by Warner and colleagues (1994), interestingly, found this to be one of the less frequent contributors to nonadherence, included by only 14% of patients in their top three reasons; nonetheless, two groups especially burdened by medication costs are the elderly and the severely and persistently mentally ill. For these groups, the cost of medications each month can easily exceed the cost of rent or even food.

Case 7

Terrance H, a 38-year-old unemployed psychiatric nurse diagnosed with schizoaffective disorder, was supported with disability payments and insured by Medicare. Living on a very limited income, he found it difficult to afford medications not covered by his insurance, particularly olanzapine (which had a more favorable side-effect profile for him than the typical neuroleptics he had previously used). Ashamed of his financial distress, he chose to discontinue the unaffordable medication rather than discuss his dilemma with his psychiatrist. When paranoid delusions about passers-by became a prominent topic of discussion in his psychotherapy, his therapist called to inform his prescribing clinician of this problem. Enrollment in a patient-assistance program procured a free supply of olanzapine for his subsequent use.

In each class of pharmaceuticals, there are more and less expensive agents. Typically, generic medications are less expensive than brand-name medications. Formulary medications are less expensive than nonformulary medications. When it is medically necessary or advisable to prescribe a more costly medication, patient-assistance programs are often available to obtain free treatment for eligible individuals. To facilitate recognition of the need for such assistance, however, the patient and clinician must engage in a dialogue, in a spirit of cooperation, and follow the practice of working collaboratively to solve problems that occur around medications.

A patient's social support system may greatly impact on how psychiatric medications are taken. Patients may sample the pills another family member is taking for similar complaints. Sometimes the "sampled" pills are used in addition to other medications they are already taking. In families where disapproval of medication is expressed as a part of stigmatization or denial of a mental disorder, the patient may choose to continue medication only secretly or to discontinue it unadvisedly. Certainly family support can almost always facilitate patient adherence; especially when the medication regimen is complicated, family support becomes even more essential.

Case 8

Elaine, a 32-year-old teacher, had long experience with bipolar disorder prior to her marriage. Her husband refused to believe that she needed lithium, which had in fact helped her remain well for a period of years, and expressed open disapproval every time he saw her take her medication. Dramatic quarrels ensued, with threats of divorce. At first, she tried to comply with his wishes. She stopped her lithium but soon thereafter experienced a resurgence of mood instability and irritability. She discussed the matter with her clinician, who discussed the available options with her. She decided, ultimately, to take her medication secretly while encouraging her husband to attend couples counseling sessions where this issue could be discussed in a venue she found less threatening.

Patients who are strongly influenced by input from their family members may find it helpful to involve the family members in their treatment. The additional information that the pharmacotherapist can gain from a spouse or other significant figure in a patient's life can make the presence of these other individuals quite valuable. The support for adherence to a medication program that a family member can contribute will many times make the difference between success and failure in treatment.

On some occasions, the major impediment to medication adherence comes from forces external to the patient and even his usual support system. A patient may be concerned that the taking of an antidepressant, for example, will impact upon the later availability of life insurance. Employees who will require a security clearance may refuse to take a medication that will be detected by a blood test.

Case 9

Ronald J, a depressed commercial pilot, benefited from treatment with fluvoxamine taken during the height of his severe symptoms. As soon as he felt moderately improved, he expressed a wish to stop the medication rather than continue for the recommended continuation phase of 6 months. "I can't return to work on this medication," he claimed, "so I have to stop it whether or not you agree."

It is necessary to acknowledge that psychiatric diagnoses still carry a stigma in our society. When a patient's realistic vocational or other needs make it impossible for pharmacotherapy to continue, the clinician can help the patient to assess his or her options. If relapse or recurrence is very likely, it may be appropriate to recommend vocational counseling and consideration of a different type of occupation. If it is reasonable to discontinue pharmacotherapy, the clinician can help the patient do this safely and recommend other ways to address the symptoms that led to treatment.

THERAPEUTIC RELATIONSHIP

A discussion of the forces that promote or undermine adherence to treatment must acknowledge the crucial role of the relationship with the prescribing clinician. Parts of the previous discussion already have touched on this, for example, in emphasizing the practical value of providing patient education in a form consistent with the patient's emotional and learning styles. I'd like to carry the discussion further by addressing how adherence to a treatment plan is affected by the working relationship and transference relationships with the prescribing clinician, the relationships with concurrent healthcare providers, and the "relationships" that the patient carries on with the pills themselves.

In a study of 82 consecutive new patients seen for an initial appointment in a psychiatric outpatient department, only 65% returned for a second appointment. One of the few predictors of return was the patient's sense of feeling "understood in the initial session and satisfied with the interview" (Zisook et al., 1978–79). Eisenthal and colleagues (1983) have measured the importance of determining the patient's "request" early in the treatment relationship and building a working alliance by restating that request to the patient for consensus. In other words, it is important to know what the patient wants in seeking treatment. Sometimes it may be very basic; at other times, it may be totally unrealistic. In today's consumer-oriented healthcare environment it is not unusual to be reminded that we clinicians are, after all, ultimately responsible to our patients to provide a service that they will find helpful. Given the growing pressure in many settings to shorten appointments, increase the interval between appointments, and narrow the role of prescribing clinician to that of a "med backup," it is all too easy to allow the prescribing role to hypertrophy at the expense of such other clinical roles as listening, empathizing, clarifying, interpreting, educating, or advising. Under such circumstances, the development of a strong and helpful working alliance becomes quite difficult.

Clinicians who function in a prescribing role must keep in mind that adherence cannot be expected from a patient who does not feel engaged in a collaborative effort. To promote the working alliance, it is helpful to identify the patient's expectations and wishes for treatment and to restate them to assure that they are correctly understood. Periodic inquiries about treatment adherence are the best way to assess whether medications are in fact being taken as directed (Rudd, 1979) and will also demonstrate the clinician's ongoing investment in the treatment process. Periodic assessments of therapeutic and adverse effects, likewise, will not only yield valuable information but will also remind the patient of the collaborative nature of the treatment relationship. The overriding value in the relationship should be to help the patient feel accepted and involved in a "subject-subject" relationship with another human being, rather than a "subject-object" relationship with an authority figure who may overlook his or her values and needs (Docherty et al., 1977). When such a relationship has been established, a clinician's questions about medication effects, symptoms, or mental status will more likely be experienced as a caring inquiry and not an intrusive interrogation.

Beyond the working alliance, each treatment relationship brings with it a set of expectations and emotions developed in earlier relationships. These transference and countertransference feelings may not be readily accessible to conscious awareness, yet can dramatically affect clinical interactions. Since a patient's contact with a pharmacotherapist may consist of relatively brief and infrequent visits, there is ample room for transferential expectations of the relationship to develop without being examined or even noted. The clinician, too, is vulnerable to projecting feelings from prior experiences onto present patients.

Case 10

I asked my patient, Deborah K, to taper and discontinue her antidepressant, citalopram, following appearance of a significant rash. Although the rash subsided, we were never certain whether it had been caused by the citalopram or by the antibiotic she had needed during the same period as the citalopram trial. Before leaving for my vacation, I started her on sertraline in hopes that it would be effective and well-tolerated. I notified her of the means for reaching me or my covering clinician if a problem arose. On my return, I received a voice mail message in which she sheepishly told me she had found sertraline ineffective after a week and therefore decided to stop it and resume the citalopram in hopes of alleviating her growing depressive symptoms. For reasons that were confusing to me, she had not tried to involve me or the covering clinician in this decision. I spoke to this patient in an angry and critical manner and was uncomfortably aware that my behavior was not typical of my usual manner with patients. Initially, I considered my anger justified because I had been left out of the patient's impulsive and unilateral decision-making process, which resulted in a potentially dangerous choice. Only through introspective analysis of my feelings, which seemed inappropriately intense, did I recall how helpless and angry I had felt a decade earlier upon learning that another patient, also named Deborah, had misused her medications, failed to contact an available clinician, and committed suicide during my vacation. Recognizing my countertransference feelings allowed me to reassess my approach. I was able to discuss the situation calmly with the patient and reach a consensus on how to proceed safely with her treatment.

Each clinician must be responsible for monitoring his or her feelings and reactions to patients and for taking care not to disrupt treatment with feelings or opinions that should be addressed outside of the treatment setting. Supervision can play a formative and ongoing role in this process. An experience with personal psychotherapy, too, can instill in the clinician a habit of looking inward and identifying personal contributions to the interpersonal field. In healthcare settings that emphasize the prescriber's role as a narrowly defined one, it is still possible (and perhaps even essential) to enhance one's effectiveness by incorporating assessment and intervention skills that can complement more traditional psychotherapeutic approaches. In one study, for example, motivational interviewing techniques were found helpful in increasing treatment adherence among outpatients with depression and cocaine dependence (Daley et al., 1998). The position of negotiation, which emphasizes understanding the other party's perspective and values and searching for mutually acceptable consensus solutions, can be a valuable approach to identifying obstacles to adherence and constructing solutions (Fisher & Ury, 1981). The role of the pharmacotherapist may even require him or her to develop powers of persuasion, given the need to enlist cooperation and follow through despite initial skepticism and a limited amount of time for collaborative discussion (Schiffman, 1999).

As a later chapter will explore, the alliance may even play a less-prominent role than the transference feelings developed in earlier interactions with other significant caregiving figures. The patient who has learned to trust will approach the prescribing clinician with a predisposition to trust while the patient who has experienced early sadistic treatment will expect a medication that is painful, harmful, and worth avoiding. Complex and dysfunctional uses of medication based on transference feelings are seen frequently in the treatment of patients with personality disorders, although they occur with the entire diagnostic spectrum of patients. The depressed patient may abstain from medications from a conviction that his prescriber has lost hope of his recovery. The anxious patient may cautiously take pill fragments rather than an entire prescribed dose, motivated by unconscious fear of becoming dependent upon the caregiver or the medication. The paranoid patient may conceal discontinuation of medication out of fear of the clinician's potential reprisals. Borderline personality disorder patients in pharmacotherapy may express unconscious feelings toward a caregiver by experiencing or using medications in a way that is symbolic of their feelings toward the clinician. Depending on the state of the transference, the medication can function as evidence of nurturance or confirmation of defectiveness or helplessness. In the struggle to assert autonomy and to avoid relinquishing control to a clinician, a borderline patient may openly or covertly avoid taking the medication as directed (Koenigsberg, 1991). Deviations from usage as directed are most likely to occur during times when transference feelings are most intense, such as times of interpersonal loss or failure, times of strong positive or negative feelings toward the clinician, or times when the patient feels the need to deny feelings of dependency on the therapist (Waldinger & Frank, 1989).

Case 11

Eileen L, a woman receiving nefazodone and naltrexone prescriptions for social phobia and for alcohol dependence in remission, confided in me that she had not been taking her naltrexone for the past 3 months. She had read about the possibility of liver damage from naltrexone and become fearful of the medication. She grew up in a sadistic and unpredictable household. I said to her, "You've come to see me each month and each month I've asked you whether the naltrexone is still effective and whether you have any side effects. Each month you say it seems effective and there are no side effects and you accept a prescription for the next month. Why haven't you told me that you weren't taking the medication?" She replied, simply, "I was afraid you'd be pissed at me." Clarification of my role and expectations, interpretation of the transference, and emphasis of our relatively solid working alliance allowed us to proceed with discontinuation of the naltrexone, which no longer seemed necessary to her now that sobriety felt well established. In addition, I was reinforcing for her that open discussion can also lead to her getting what she thinks is correct as well as expressing confidence in her ability to abstain without the assistance of medications.

The patient's relationship with the medication and his adherence to a treatment plan can also be affected by interactions with other significant figures in his life. The patient's relationship with his medications comprises to a great extent displaced feelings. These feelings may be ones held toward the prescribing clinician and/or toward family members. As Smith (1989) has noted,

> These displacements provide much of the dynamic basis of nonadherence. A patient who gets mad at a parent, for example, might stop taking pills in an effort to punish his parent. He may have little insight into his motives, noting only that at times (of anger) the taste of the medication is physically revolting. A paranoid patient may experience a pill as the concrete manifestation of an authority's wish to do him harm. So, too, the medication can sometimes become the vehicle of a patient's transference of hate toward either caregiver. When this occurs, an attempted or completed suicide can be the tragic result. (pp. 92–93)

Case 12

Early in my career, I was asked to examine a persistently ill schizophrenic patient, Arnold M, a long-term resident of the state hospital whose treatment with trifluoperazine was causing a severe parkinsonian tremor. I was covering for my colleague, Dr. Adams, a gentle and empathic clinician who was very attentive to his patient's needs. Pressed for time, I examined the patient somewhat perfunctorily and prescribed the appropriate dose of benztropine (Cogentin). The next day, despite what I thought to be improvement of the tremor, Mr. M cornered me in the hall and plaintively said, "I don't want to take your Cogentin. I prefer the Cogentin that Dr. Adams gives me."

Even though we may be functioning primarily as "prescribers" or "med backups,"[2] we must continue to draw upon the full range of clinical skills including assessment, formulation, active listening, empathy, and support. Attention to transference and to possible distortions in communication, particularly in a treatment where dialogue and exchange of information has been the norm, will facilitate adherence to a treatment regimen.

For many patients, one of their most significant human interactions is that which takes place with the psychotherapist, who is increasingly rarely also the prescribing psychiatrist. The psychotherapist is in a powerful position to strengthen medication adherence or to undermine it. Of great importance to the treatment, therefore, is collaboration between the prescribing clinician and the psychotherapist, a topic discussed at greater length elsewhere (Sederer et al., 1998) as well as elsewhere in this book. Suffice it to note here that the prescribing clinician should share with the psychotherapist sufficient information about the diagnosis, treatment options, rationale for the choices made, and plans for treatment to allow the psychotherapist to support the pharmacotherapy in a knowledgeable manner. Similarly, the pharmacotherapist needs to have some appreciation of what the psychotherapist is doing in that component of the treatment. As emphasized by Balon (1999, p. 23), "In good collaborative treatment, the therapist takes an active stance about medication, knows the common therapeutic and side effects of medication, reminds the patient

---

[2] Use of this term here does not condone the notion, currently widespread, that psychiatrists can function primarily as prescribers in clinical settings where psychotherapy is assigned to less-costly clinicians. The apparent convenience and possible cost-savings (a disputed point) associated with this specialized psychiatric role may obscure an important clinical and risk-management concern, which is that even when psychiatrists feel they are serving only as a "med backup" they remain accountable for understanding their patients' clinical difficulties and treatment plans in a broader way and must do so in order to prescribe rationally.

TABLE 4.1. Obstacles and Interventions for Enhancing
Pharmacotherapy Adherence

Pharmacotherapy adherence obstacle	Suggested intervention(s)
Level of distress and motivation	
Too little	Assess suitability of diagnosis and symptoms for pharmacotherapy
	Assess which symptoms are most important to patient
	Assess comorbid diagnoses
Denial	Assess level of denial
Externalization	Assess patient's competence to accept or refuse treatment
Medication effects	
Side effects	Choose medication with tolerable side effect profile
	Choose medication with side effects tolerable to specific patient treated
	Educate patient about side effects to the degree appropriate, in appropriate manner
	Monitor clinical and laboratory parameters of side effects
Therapeutic effects	Assess and monitor therapeutic effects of medication
Treatment accessibility	
Chaotic life, lack of routine	Address patient's life routine
Discontinuous care due to system	Assess continuity of care
Unaffordable care	Assess cost of treatment, including medication
External pressures against treatment	Assess social support system
	Assess effects of employer or other external sources of potential influence
Treatment relationship	
Working alliance	Assess working alliance
Countertransference	Assess countertransference
Transference	Assess transference
"Relationship" to medications	Assess relationship to medications
Role of concurrent psychotherapist	Assess influence of concurrent psychotherapist

of the need for faithful adherence, and is prepared to be an advocate for the patient when problems arise in pharmacotherapy."

CONCLUSION

Although we await ever-more specific and tolerable medications, we can nonetheless increase the effectiveness of treatment by paying more attention to the factors that affect adherence to treatment and the means at our disposal for addressing them (see Table 4.1). Attention must be paid to each patient's level of distress and motivation, to the effects and side effects of medications, to the accessibility and context of treatment, and to the therapeutic relationship with the prescriber. For each area of concern, specific techniques are available to address adherence problems. In this way, adherence will be enhanced and the medications we prescribe will be more likely to deliver their potential benefits to our patients.

CHAPTER FIVE

Transference and Countertransference

Michael D. Jibson, MD, PhD

Case 1

Ms. A is a 35-year-old single woman who presented herself to Dr. D's medication clinic for evaluation of depression. She was well dressed, professional, and quite attractive. She reported having become increasingly depressed since the termination of a long-term relationship with her fiancé, leaving her without his companionship, with little prospect for the family she wanted, and with a significant financial burden. During the initial interview, she gave terse answers to all the clinical questions, volunteered no additional information, and made it clear that her only goal was to receive a prescription for antidepressant medications, explaining that her financial situation did not allow the possibility of simultaneous psychotherapy. Her demeanor was tense and somewhat angry. She met all criteria for major depression, was not actively suicidal, and had no significant medical problems. Dr. D, a married man of 45, discussed the risks and benefits of a specific medication, gave her a prescription, and arranged for follow-up within a reasonable period of time.

Ms. A was compliant in taking the medication, but showed only modest improvement. She complained about the limited effectiveness of the medication, but always agreed to continue it. She remained tense and angry, and avoided Dr. D's repeated attempts to engage her in a broader discussion of her problems. Dr. D felt increasingly defensive and frustrated. Reviewing the case at a weekly meeting with colleagues, he became aware of his personal issues regarding her choices of relationship, career, and family, which he believed to be fundamentally flawed, and therefore inevitably disappointing. Only after he recognized his own latent anger at her choices was he able to make the obvious interpretation to her, "You always seem more angry than depressed, perhaps that needs to be addressed as well." As she walked out of the office, she asked him, in reference to herself, "Don't you get tired of all these depressed people?" She quickly retracted the question, saying that it was not fair of her to ask. Dr. D was struck for the first time by the depth of her vulnerability in presenting herself to the clinic. Noting the limited time, he offered reassurance regarding the reality of her pain and the potential benefits of treatment. The following sessions included brief exploration of a number of personal issues, which proved to be helpful in resolving her depression.

Transference refers to the displacement of feelings, thoughts, and attitudes from significant past relationships to a current situation. Although this concept was originally intended to describe a specific phenomenon within psychoanalysis, it is clear that transference occurs in all personal interactions. Indeed, all aspects of relationships throughout life are strongly influenced by past experience. The capacity for trust, friendship, and love, as well as style of interaction, personal expectations, emotional availability, and tolerance for ambiguity in relationships are closely tied to early experience.

As therapeutic techniques and theories have developed, it has become clear that transference feelings do not derive purely from unconscious drives and conflicts, but rather occur in conjunction with more appropriate responses to the realities of a current situation. Every patient-therapist encounter involves not only the history that each brings to the meeting, but also the realities of the relationship between them. Thus, most transference feelings will be triggered by, or relate to, some aspect of the actual situation. Conversely, even feelings that are clearly appropriate to the current situation are determined to some degree by transference.

Within the clinical setting, transference feelings are especially prominent. In this context, transference may be broadly defined as the feelings of the patient toward the psychiatrist. By extension, the patient may have feelings about the medications prescribed, other forms of treatment in use, the clinic setting, or the larger institution in which treatment occurs.

Case 2

Dr. F looked with annoyance at Mr. C's name on her afternoon schedule. He was always late for their standing monthly appointment, arriving five minutes before the end of their 20-minute session, then requiring the full 20 minutes for her to drag out of him the basic information about his response to the medication. The remainder of her day was always tightly booked, and there was no opportunity to get back on schedule. She typically responded by attempting to cut short his visit, asking only cursory questions, and quickly refilling his medication. An anxious man, with significant avoidant traits, Mr. C endured the sessions with difficulty, but was otherwise rigid in his compliance with treatment recommendations. Dr. F suspected that he was trying to minimize the therapeutic intimacy developing during their brief visits. She asked him on this occasion if the sessions made him nervous. He clearly became more anxious in response to the question, but assured her that he had no such feelings, and attempted to hurry through the session by giving even more curt answers than usual.

After he left, Dr. F commented on his tardiness to the receptionist, who pointed out that he rode a city bus to the sessions, which ran on an hourly schedule. His only options were to arrive 45 minutes early and sit in the waiting area with a dozen other people, or arrive 15 minutes late. Too shy to ask for a different time, Mr. C had chosen the least anxiety-provoking of his options. At the following visit, Dr. F suggested a different time for their appointments, to which the patient agreed, and which resulted in his consistent arrival on time.

In this case, an element of reality, the bus schedule, interacted with the patient's high level of anxiety and avoidance to create a specific problem. Dr. F correctly identified that there was an issue to discuss and that it involved the patient's psychopathology, but the problem could only be addressed when the real situation was also brought into the picture.

Countertransference refers to the feelings of the psychiatrist toward the patient. These feelings were originally conceptualized as the therapist's own unresolved conflicts, which were displaced onto the patient. It is now widely accepted that countertransference is predominantly a reflection of the patient's feelings and behavior, and the psychiatrist's reaction to them, rather than representing a manifestation of the psychiatrist's own unconscious pathology. The psychiatrist is likely to respond to such factors as the patient's unique interpersonal style, symptoms, coping strategies, attitudes toward medication and other treatments, and degree of treatment compliance. As such, countertransference feelings may communicate to the psychiatrist important information about the patient. Countertransference feelings may, however, also originate exclusively within the psychiatrist, whose attitudes, thoughts, and feelings about specific diagnoses, medications, psychotherapy, the clinic setting, and the larger system in which the patient is seen will also have an impact on the therapeutic relationship.

Like transference, countertransference phenomena are prominent in the medication clinic, and must be understood and addressed for effective treatment to be provided. This chapter will consider the ways in which transference and countertransference feelings have both a positive and a negative impact on the medication management of psychiatric symptoms, and will explore strategies for incorporation of these concepts into effective clinical care.

TRANSFERENCE

Transference may be broadly divided into two types, positive and negative. Positive transference refers to feelings of idealization, admiration, respect, attraction, love, and so forth. These feelings tend to draw the patient toward the psychiatrist, facilitate their work together, and increase the likelihood of the patient's compliance with treatment.

Negative transference, in contrast, includes feelings of hostility, anger, resentment, devaluation, hatred, and rejection. These feelings tend to drive the patient away from the psychiatrist, and are often associated with poor treatment compliance and response.

The Psychiatrist

The most often noted object of both positive and negative transference is the psychiatrist. In the medication clinic even patients' immediate response to the psychiatrist may be determined as much by their expectations and predilections as by the psychiatrist's personality and interpersonal style. Patients rarely enter a psychiatry clinic without significant expectations, fears, and fantasies about the psychiatrist they will meet and the care they will receive. In addition, media portrayals, accounts of friends and family, and interactions with prior care providers have a powerful impact on the patient's expectations. The patient's experience of the initial encounter with the psychiatrist will be strongly colored by these expectations.

Under the best of circumstances, a positive transference will begin to develop toward the psychiatrist within the initial visit. Specific patient responses to the initial interview, such as confidence and trust, a sense of validation regarding the presenting complaint, and feeling nurtured and cared for, will enhance the therapeutic relationship and strengthen the patient's commitment to treatment. Although some of the patient's initial reaction to the psychiatrist is driven by outside factors, much of this early response is based in reality. Early positive transference will be enhanced by a professional appearance, observance of standard social conventions, empathic listening, patient education, patient involvement in decision making, adherence to scheduled appointment times, a prompt, focused response to telephone calls, and courteous, efficient support staff. By contrast, early negative transference may arise if the patient perceives that the psychiatrist is disorganized, odd, rude, uninterested, careless, dismissive, or authoritarian (Table 5.1).

Case 3

Mr. W was a 65-year-old married executive and engineer, recently contemplating retirement from the successful high-technology company he founded two decades before high-tech was in vogue. He had recently been diagnosed with prostate cancer, denied his obvious anxiety about it, and was promptly referred by his urologist to the psychiatry clinic. Throughout his life, personal feelings had never been considered a legitimate basis for decision making, and he took pride in his ability to disregard them. He believed, however, that the opinion of experts, particularly experts outside his own field, should be trusted, and on that basis he made the initial call to the clinic, and appeared on time for his evaluation.

Dr. N was a young man of conservative upbringing and values. He appeared at the waiting room door on time, neatly groomed and conventionally dressed in slacks, collared shirt, and necktie.

He began, "Mr. W? How do you do? I am Dr. N. My office is right over here, please come this way."

TABLE 5.1. Interaction of External and Internal Factors in Positive and Negative Transference Feelings Experienced by the Patient toward the Psychiatrist and the Medication Early in Treatment

	External (real) issues	Transference feelings
	Positive factors	
Psychiatrist	Professional appearance	Confidence and trust
	Observance of social conventions	Validation of symptoms and distress
	Empathic listening	Nurtured
	Patient education	Cared for
	Patient involvement in decision making	Educated
	Adherence to scheduled appointment times	
	Prompt, focused response to telephone calls	
	Courteous, efficient support staff	
Medication	Highly effective	Benevolent gift
	Favorable side-effect profile	Healing remedy
	Easy to use	Useful tool
	Rapid response	Validation of suffering
		Source of hope
		Transitional object
	Negative factors	
Psychiatrist	Disorganized	Distrust
	Odd behavior, grooming, or dress	Lack of confidence
	Rude interactions	Dismissed symptoms and distress
	Uninterested in patient	Rejected
	Careless	Disregarded
	Dismissive of complaints	Demeaned
	Authoritarian	Confused
Medication	Limited effectiveness	Crutch
	Unfavorable side effects	Artificial treatment
	Difficult to remember	Poison
	Gradual response	Deny or avoid real issues
		Minimize interaction with therapist

Mr. W entered and glanced nervously at the couch along one wall, commenting, "You really do have a couch."

Noticing his discomfort, Dr. N responded with a smile, "Yes, it's more convenient than bringing in a bunch of chairs when I meet with families."

Mr. W focused closely on the issue at hand, his impending surgery and the urologist's concerns about his anxiety. He answered all the questions forthrightly, and with matter-of-fact emotional disconnection.

Dr. N discussed the impact of anxiety on routine surgery, emphasizing somatic effects, and concurred with the surgeon's concern. He outlined several treatment options, then recommended a specific medication. The patient agreed, already appearing less anxious.

As he left the office, he commented, "Thank you, this was a lot different than I thought it would be."

Mr. W's anxiety was heightened by his concern over what would happen during his psychiatric evaluation. Dr. N's appearance and demeanor were much like those of professionals in other fields, and so tended to put Mr. W at ease, as did his focus on the issue at hand.

As treatment continues, the patient's initial perceptions and feelings about the psychiatrist will be refined, but in only a few cases will they be rejected altogether. Added to the initial impressions will be additional transference reactions arising more particularly from the patient's personal issues, but continuing to be influenced by the realities of the situation. It is during this second phase of treatment that issues of communication, control, and compliance become most prominent.

Case 4

Ms. H was a 23-year-old woman with panic disorder, referred to Dr. P in the outpatient clinic following a brief series of panic attacks. She responded well to medication, which had few side effects, and posed no obvious problems for her. During the course of her treatment, she asked incessant questions about the medication, its long-term effects, studies conducted on persons of her gender and age, and so forth. She also constantly sought reassurance regarding Dr. P's qualifications to treat her, asking about his acquaintance with research in the area of panic disorder, number of patients with a similar diagnosis he had treated, and familiarity with the literature on her medication. She demanded more and more frequent appointments, until she was being seen weekly for 30-minute sessions. Dr. P frequently noted Ms. H's significant narcissistic traits, and assumed that her demands occurred exclusively in that context.

Because of her escalating need for treatment, Dr. P suggested a transfer to a clinic which offered a more intensive level of care, to which the patient responded with vehement opposition. Only then did she reveal that she had developed a significant erotic transference to Dr. P, which led her to seek ever-more frequent contact with him, and was now threatened by the prospect of transfer.

Ms. H's medication response was overshadowed by her transference issues, first her narcissistic demand for impossibly detailed and personalized information, then her erotic transference. Her positive transference initially enhanced treatment, but Dr. P failed to recognize the erotic quality of Ms. H's feelings, and therefore did not respond to them appropriately. Ultimately, the problems created by the transference became more pronounced than the benefits of the medication, and nearly destroyed the treatment altogether.

A unique variant of positive transference has been characterized as an "idealizing transference." This concept was introduced by Heinz Kohut (1968), who suggested that developing personalities need to receive attention, love, and admiration from the very people who are most important to them. While this is readily apparent in reference to children seeking positive attention from parents, it is also operative in the clinical setting. The importance to the patient of attention from the idealized physician, the value of the title "Doctor," the status of the attending physician, and the medical authority of the psychiatrist should not be underestimated. These can be useful tools in establishing a positive therapeutic relationship, and the denial to patients of the physician's time and attention may be experienced as a personal blow. Similarly, if these factors are wielded in such a way as to make the patient feel demeaned or less important, they can be enormously destructive.

Case 5

Dr. T was a senior psychiatric resident working in the university outpatient clinic. A capable physician, she looked forward to graduation in a few months. She was quite distressed, therefore, to find the case assigned to her for evaluation that morning to be quickly getting out of hand. The patient, Mr. G, was a 22-year-old man with schizophrenia, brought in by his family, who had recently moved to the area. Although Mr. G appeared stable on his current medications, he was not working or going to school, and spent most of his time at home watching television.

The family seemed angry from the time they walked into the clinic. They expressed dissatisfaction with Dr. T's general concurrence with the previous treatment. They were unhappy with the frequency of visits Dr. T recommended. They demanded a series of aggressive diagnostic tests, some of which had been done elsewhere, and some of which were not clinically appropriate. They also stated that they expected to have the final word on all treatment decisions. Dr. T patiently spent additional time with them, attempted to share information on antipsychotic medications, discussed with them the selection of diagnostic tests, and reviewed the legal requirements for informed consent. The family became more angry and dissatisfied than ever. Feeling defeated and a failure, Dr. T asked the attending psychiatrist, Dr. M, to step in. The family calmed immediately upon Dr. M's arrival. She presented precisely the same information and perspective as the resident, but this time it was accepted gratefully. After the visit, Dr. T was defensive and hurt, knowing that she had tried to do everything the attending had succeeded at doing.

The presence of the attending psychiatrist, perceived as the "final authority," was the critical element for Mr. G's family. They were angry at their perception of not receiving attention from the attending physician, and chose to put little trust in the resident, Dr. T, despite the reality of her competence. It was not the actions of the attending, but her identity and role, to which they responded.

Response to Diagnosis

Patients, as well as physicians, attach meaning to diagnoses. A patient's response to a diagnosis of bipolar disorder, for example, is likely to differ significantly from that to narcissistic personality disorder. In some cases, such as major depressive disorder, massive public campaigns not only heighten awareness of the diagnosis, but also shape public perception of its meaning. Understandably, patients are more accepting of diagnoses that carry no implication of responsibility or blame. Similarly, patients are resistant to diagnoses implying that a change in attitude or perception is all that is required for effective treatment.

This is not to suggest that resort to biological reductionism is a beneficial direction for all patients. While it may be helpful to persuade a depressed patient that she is not expected to "just get over it," to suggest to the borderline patient that his rapid mood swings are merely the manifestation of a "chemical imbalance" is not therapeutically prudent. Patient education, coupled with attention to the patient's perceptions of the diagnosis, are most likely to yield positive results.

Case 6

Ms. P is a 29-year-old woman, newly referred to Dr. H's clinic. She had received a variety of diagnoses over the several years that she had been treated for mood swings and repeated suicide attempts. Among them were dysthymic disorder, posttraumatic stress disorder, substance abuse, major depressive disorder, eating disorder, impulse control disorder NOS, and most recently bipolar II disorder.

Dr. H obtained a history of a lifetime pattern of mood instability, mostly involving sudden, brief mood swings. She had chronic feelings of emptiness. She responded with anger and despair to real or threatened abandonment. She used her chronic suicidality as a means of distress reduction and manipulation of her environment. Dr. H was persuaded that the most appropriate diagnosis was borderline personality disorder. Dr. H sat down with the patient to discuss diagnosis. "I understand that you have been frustrated by all the diagnoses and treatments that you have received over the years. In reviewing your history, several patterns emerge which suggest that the most appropriate diagnosis may be borderline personality disorder."

Ms. P was angry and defensive. "You're saying it's just all in my head, that it's all my fault. Why did the last doctor tell me I had bipolar disorder, if it was really a personality disorder?"

Dr. H remained calm, and gently leaned forward to emphasize his points. He spoke quietly, but distinctly. "Much of your history is tied to mood swings, and that suggests bipolar disorder, but that diagnosis is too narrow to describe the full range of what you have experienced. When a person's distress has lasted so long, and arises from so many parts of life, when it involves not just moods, but relationships, coping style, and even self-concept, a broader diagnosis is more likely to lead to useful treatment. These difficulties arise from a combination of what is happening in the brain with what is happening in your world. Your diagnosis and your treatment need to cover both."

The resulting discussion defused much of Ms. P's initial anger at the diagnosis, and was able to focus attention on the multidisciplinary treatment most likely to be beneficial.

Few things are as difficult to tell a patient as a diagnosis of personality disorder. In this instance, Dr. H focused on the positive aspects of having a correct diagnosis. These include a reduction in Ms. P's frustration with multiple diagnoses, and the benefits of having a diagnostic category broad enough to encompass the full range of the patient's difficulties. This broader diagnostic focus allowed a broader treatment plan, as well, with immediate benefit.

Transference to Medications and Other Therapies

Most patients come into the clinic with specific feelings about medications, psychotherapy, and different types of therapists. These feelings may be strongly tied to the present circumstances, or may be the product of past experiences, fears, preconceptions, philosophical stance, and fantasies (Dewan, 1992; Goldhamer, 1983; Waldinger & Frank, 1989).

Few patients coming into a clinic are unaware of the existence of medications, and some medications are widely known. The two-edged sword of publicity has the effect of communicating to individuals that their suffering may be a treatable psychiatric condition, that medications may be effective, and that the stigma of mental illness is misplaced. But publicity also highlights exceptional cases of physician misconduct, fringe-group opinions regarding treatment, and unsubstantiated fears of medication side effects or abuse. Most patients come into the clinic with some feelings about medication, and much of their initial response to a medication recommendation will be determined by those preconceived ideas.

Positive transference may cause the patient to see the medication as a benevolent gift, a healing remedy, a useful tool, a validation of suffering, a source of hope, or a transitional object. In this case, the act of accepting the medicine is itself therapeutic, and each dose of the medication is a positive step in the patient's mind. These feelings will support medication compliance and strengthen the alliance with the prescriber.

They may also extend too far, into the realm of unrealistic expectations and false hope. It is not surprising in this context to find placebo response rates up to 30% for disorders such as major depression.

Negative transference toward medications may lead patients to see them as a demeaning crutch, artificial treatment, poison, or means of avoiding dealing with the "real issues." In these cases, patients may focus on side effects, which they see as evidence of harm. Compliance will be poor, and the relationship with the psychiatrist will deteriorate (Table 5.1).

In general, it is better to address these preconceptions at the beginning of the therapeutic relationship, rather than after a problem develops. It is appropriate to ask about the patient's preferences before discussion of treatment options, and perhaps even before the diagnostic evaluation. If the psychiatrist has a strong predilection for specific treatments, these should be explicitly stated at the outset. A neutral stance, emphasizing the value of different modes of treatment, is especially helpful. Patient education is also useful to create an appropriate environment for consideration of these issues.

Transference feelings regarding medication may also emerge later in treatment, as the degree of medication effectiveness, presence or absence of side effects, or the realities of daily compliance become clearer. Positive transference may be enhanced by an excellent treatment response, lack of side effects, and ease of medication use, while negative transference will be accentuated by the opposite developments. Patients also tend to be highly attuned to the psychiatrist's response to these issues as they arise. Additional subjects of concern, not obvious at the outset of treatment, may also come into play. Control issues may become prominent, as the patient either complies or fails to comply with dosage and frequency of medication, displays a propensity for unauthorized medication adjustment, or engages in clear manipulation of the treatment situation. The ability and willingness of the patient to communicate with the psychiatrist also becomes more pronounced as treatment progresses.

Case 7

Mrs. K was a 68-year-old cancer patient, referred for treatment of depression. She had a distant history of one prior episode of depression, for which she had received no specific treatment. She noted a decline in her mood shortly after starting cancer chemotherapy last year. She was started on an antidepressant, and was invited to a support group, but had not found the initial dosage of medication particularly effective, and did not feel that "just talking to people" would be helpful. She consistently told her doctor that the antidepressant was "fine," because she did not expect the medication to be helpful, but did not want to disappoint the doctor. Only when she broke down in tears during a visit with her oncologist did it become clear that additional exploration of her expectations and evaluation of antidepressant treatment was in order.

Mrs. K had certain expectations regarding the meaning and utility of medications and psychotherapy, both of which interfered with the treatment. Only when sufficient opportunity to explore those assumptions arose was she able to effectively use any form of treatment.

Transference to the Clinic Setting

Just as patients bring preconceptions and expectations to the individual psychiatrist, so they bring them to the clinic or institution where they come to see you. Large university medical centers tend to engender feelings of competence and professionalism. At the same time, some patients experience the staff as cold and aloof, and may fear that they will be used for training or research purposes. Health maintenance organizations and managed care programs can be viewed in a positive light, focusing on primary prevention of illness and prompt, effective care, or they may be taken as spendthrift bureaucracies interested only in cutting costs. Solo private practitioners may be seen as experienced, independent, and caring physicians delivering individualized care, or they may be seen as isolated, with limited resources, and inherently resistant to making appropriate referrals. The patient's perceptions will be strongly affected by these preexisting assumptions, whether or not they represent reality. These should be identified when they arise, and explored promptly and sensitively.

Case 8

Dr. V had worked for several years in a solo practice office, augmented with several hours of contract work at a large HMO. A major source of referrals to her practice was the emergency service at a nearby university hospital, which used community physicians to supplement a relatively small faculty. Dr. V took care to assure consistency in her practice, despite the variety of clinical settings in which she worked. During one week, she encountered a series of three patients with major depressive disorder, and discussed with each of them the relative benefits of psychotherapy and antidepressant medication.

Mr. B had classic symptoms of depression beginning after a series of disappointments in his work. He saw Dr. V in the HMO where he had coverage for the past year. Dr. V suggested the antidepressant AD, which had been on the market a little over a year, and with which she had good results. She also suggested that a brief course of psychotherapy would be appropriate. Mr. B reacted with skepticism and mild anger.

"I know how these HMOs work," he said, "I didn't really expect that I would get a full course of therapy."

Ms. J was seen in Dr. V's private office with a recurrent depressive episode after the birth of her second child. She had discontinued her antidepressant medication two years before, despite her previous psychiatrist's recommendation that she continue. Concerned about her potential for noncompliance, and the changes in her life heralded by the birth of a second child, Dr. V recommended antidepressant AD and a brief course of psychotherapy.

Ms. J was skeptical of the need for psychotherapy, and commented to her husband, "I think Dr. V just needs to fill hours in her practice."

Mr. F presented himself to the university hospital psychiatric service with symptoms of depression in the context of a marital separation. Dr. V was called in to see him, and recommended antidepressant AD and a brief course of psychotherapy.

Never having heard of AD, Mr. F responded, "You university doctors are always trying out experimental therapies on patients. Well, I'm not your guinea pig."

Dr. V reflected with mild amusement on the diversity of reactions. Later that week, she received a review of her pattern of treatment recommendations from the HMO, showing that 60% of her patients were treated with medications only, while 40% received medications plus psychotherapy. Noting that the ratio in her private practice was reversed—60% psychotherapy plus medication and 40% medication only—she was surprised that the two populations from which the patients were taken were so different.

Each of Dr. V's patients brought a set of assumptions that had a greater impact on their reactions to the treatment recommendations than did the realities of the situation. Dr. V, however, also experienced a blind spot in her mistaken perception of complete objectivity in offering treatment recommendations. This brings us to our discussion of countertransference.

COUNTERTRANSFERENCE

As with the patient's transference, the psychiatrist brings both positive and negative expectations and assumptions to the therapeutic encounter. Positive countertransference may include feelings of beneficence, generosity, acceptance, acknowledgement of pain, and nurturing. Negative countertransference may include anger, coercion, passivity, rejection, dismissal of complaints, denial of empathy, and rigidity. To an even greater degree than is the case with patients' transference, countertransference is a response to the patient and the real circumstance of treatment, and is not primarily a manifestation of the psychiatrist's personal issues. It would not be accurate, however, to suggest that the psychiatrist is free of assumptions and expectations in the clinical setting.

Case 9

Mrs. S was a 65-year-old woman who had been treated for major depression disorder by Dr. R over several years, with good results. She was on maintenance medication therapy when she was diagnosed with ovarian cancer, already widely metastatic. Her mood declined slightly, and Dr. R made an appropriate adjustment in her medication.

In an effort to express his understanding of her situation, Dr. R observed, "I wish I had more to offer than just medications; I don't really feel that I am serving you very well with just a prescription."

She responded, "But you are. The medication is making it possible for me to keep going and doing the things I want to do."

Dr. R assumed in this case that medications represented a limitation on therapy, that Mrs. S was inadequately treated, and that she expected additional modes of treatment. He responded to his own feelings of hopelessness and guilt regarding his perception of the limited range of benefits of medication by seeking the patient's reassurance. His guilt was accentuated when he realized the role reversal he brought about by placing the patient in the position of offering him support. In fact, the patient did not expect more than the psychiatrist and medication were able to provide.

Clinician Response to the Patient

Psychiatrists prefer some patients to others. The basis on which the individual practitioner selects the patient population with whom to work includes a variety of factors, most of them personal, and some of them unconscious. Secondary factors, such as training, previous experience, clinic expectations, contractual arrangements, and financial issues also enter the picture.

Although it is rarely possible to elucidate the reasons, both conscious and unconscious, for a psychiatrist's preferences among patients, it is possible to define many of the qualities of those patients. Preferences based on age are largely institutionalized; child and geriatric psychiatry are now recognized subspecialties. Preferences regarding diagnosis may affect the physician's choice of workplace; patient populations in community mental health, Veterans Affairs, solo private practice, and managed care contract clinics will be skewed in predictable directions. It is both acceptable and desirable for psychiatrists to recognize and acknowledge their patterns of patient preference, and to adjust their practices accordingly.

Individual patients also arouse specific feelings within the physician. Although these may represent issues unique to the individual psychiatrist, more often they are a direct response to the patient's appearance, interpersonal style, psychopathology, and coping strategies. The intensity and acceptability of countertransference feelings to a certain patient are expected to vary widely among clinicians, but the basic feelings aroused in specific clinical encounters are more predictable. Thus, while most psychiatrists experience anger when flagrantly manipulated by a patient, the intensity of anger, degree of perceived impairment to treatment, and willingness to continue working with the patient will be different for each practitioner.

Clinician Response to the Diagnosis

Psychiatrists have preferred diagnoses. Some of these represent trends in the profession at large (e.g., the now-passé "schizophrenogenic parent"), while others are more individual (e.g., bipolar vs. borderline personality disorders). These preferences are based on professional experience and training, personal philosophy, and other less obvious factors. If not countered, these personal tendencies may overshadow more pertinent clinical factors. Many institutionalized efforts are directed to this issue, such as DSM-IV, structured clinical interviews for diagnosis (SCIDs), and peer review. Additionally, individual practitioners have an obligation to maintain the integrity of their diagnostic and case formulations by constantly examining their diagnostic tendencies, and by following established criteria in these areas.

Case 10

Ms. L was a 52-year-old woman with a ten-year history of major depressive disorder, refractory to medications, ECT, and cognitive-behavioral therapy. As her distress was prolonged, Ms. L came to treat the mental health profession with skepticism bordering on cynical contempt. She was angry about her continued inability to function, her dependency on family for social support, and the need to see physicians for continued certification of disability to avoid loss of insurance coverage and maintenance of at least limited income. She felt increasingly hopeless, made two suicide attempts, and continued to harbor suicidal thoughts, which she experienced as a promise of relief. She feared that her family would "burn out" and abandon her. She presented herself, at her insurer's insistence, to Dr. A at a university clinic for yet another evaluation. During the initial interview, she was short-tempered and sarcastic, even when discussing her suicide attempts. She was dismissive of suggested therapies, and made it clear that she simply wanted to complete the evaluation and leave. Although her history showed conclusively that she functioned well personally, socially, and professionally prior to the onset of depression ten years ago, Dr. A was skeptical of this information, and made a diagnosis of borderline personality disorder. He recommended that the focus of treatment shift from depression to coping skills, and that the patient be dropped from her medication clinic and be placed on a "borderline track."

Although Ms. L had developed many features typical of borderline personality disorder since the onset of her depression, she did not meet the criteria for that diagnosis, and was unlikely to benefit from treatment focused on that secondary pathology. Dr. A's excessive focus on character pathology led to an incorrect diagnosis and suboptimal treatment.

Countertransference feelings also serve a useful function in diagnosis and psychodynamic formulation. Specific patient behaviors, even when subtly presented, may arouse near-universal reactions in their care providers. Among the most common feelings suggestive of specific patient dynamics are anger, defensiveness, hopelessness, boredom, fear, narcissism, sexual arousal, and rescue fantasies. Although not truly universal, these feelings often signal the presence of manipulation, anger, hopelessness, personal disconnection, paranoia or aggression, idealization, seductiveness, or dependency. Common relationships between specific countertransference feelings and patient symptoms or behaviors are outlined in Table 5.2. Attention to these countertransference feelings as they arise will aid the astute clinician in understanding the patient.

Specific diagnoses may have meaning to the psychiatrist, or may simply arouse specific feelings. A diagnosis may be regarded as routine, reassuring, readily correctable, frustrating, hopeless, or annoying. Some diagnoses are more exciting than others, a fact rarely missed by patients, who are highly motivated to appear as interesting and involving to their clinicians as possible. The psychiatrist's demeanor will be strongly af-

TABLE 5.2. Diagnostic Possibilities to Be Considered in Response to Countertransference Feelings

Countertransference feeling	Possible patient symptom
Anger	Manipulation
Boredom	Personal disconnection
Defensiveness	Anger, hostility
Fear	Paranoia, aggression
Hopelessness	Hopelessness
Narcissism	Idealization
Rescue fantasies	Dependency
Sexual arousal	Seductiveness

fected by these feelings, as will the likelihood that a specific diagnosis will be attached to a patient.

Case 11

Ms. Q was a 28-year-old woman with a long-standing diagnosis of borderline personality disorder, seeing Dr. E through community mental health. She had made little progress with a combination of individual therapy and medications. Her sessions had fallen into a routine of acceptance of a moderate level of pathology. At one medication session, she mentioned that she sometimes felt as though she were a different person, and had even toyed with the idea of changing her name. Dr. E responded with immediate interest, sat up, and fired a series of screening questions.

"Do you really feel like a different person? Have you ever called yourself by a different name? Do you have lapses in memory? Have you ever found yourself somewhere without knowing how you got there? Are there large blank spots in your childhood memories?"

Responding to the sudden interest from her psychiatrist, Ms Q managed to think of examples of each of these phenomena. Soon their sessions were focused on dissociative experiences and Dr. E changed the diagnosis to dissociative identity disorder, a diagnosis about which he had read, but had never seen or treated. The patient showed temporary improvement, but soon split the treatment team into those who focused on dissociative symptoms, and those who saw primarily borderline dynamics.

Ms. Q quite predictably responded to Dr. E's interest in dissociative phenomena by adjusting her symptoms accordingly. It soon became clear that this was a blind alley, with negative consequences in her long-term treatment.

Clinician Response to Medication

Positive and negative countertransference toward medications are also powerful determinants of treatment decisions (Goldhamer, 1983). The psychiatrist may believe that somatic treatments are "real medicine," in contrast to the vagaries of psychotherapy, or may have the opposite feeling, that the too-frequent prescription of medication is selling out to the demands of the medical marketplace, leaving little room to address the "real issues." These feelings will invariably be communicated to the patient.

Similarly, choice of medication class and of individual medication is driven by factors not limited to published placebo-controlled studies. Prior experience, anecdotal evidence, the observation of subtle trends in treatment response, subliminal aspects of the patient's presentation, and the unconscious response of the clinician to the patient all contribute to the making of decisions. This process should become increasingly effective with the acquisition of experience and constitute the essence of clinical wisdom.

Masquerading as clinical wisdom is the sclerosis of habit and rote. It is sometimes difficult for the individual clinician to distinguish between the increasing comfort that comes with clinical experience and that which simply signals growing rigidity. Every psychiatrist must be on guard against this tendency; hence participation in peer review, continuing education, and maintenance of an open mind are essential.

Clinician Response to the Clinic Setting

The nature of the relationship between an individual patient and a psychiatrist is in large part defined by the clinical setting in which they see each other. In general, structured clinics set clear guidelines for the role of psychiatrists and other professionals working there. The psychiatrist's role may be limited to prescribing, or may include team interactions, supervision of other professionals, or the option of doing brief or long-term psychotherapy. Even in a private practice, where few limitations on the selection of therapies may be in place, limitations of insurance coverage, patient finances, psychiatrist training and experience, or physical facility may have an impact on treatment options. In general it is better to discuss limitations on the therapeutic relationship at the beginning of treatment, rather than to ignore them, accept them as implicit, or wait until a problem arises.

Psychiatrists' feelings toward the clinical setting in which they work also have an impact on their relationships with individual patients. If a psychiatrist is dissatisfied with the management or operation of the clinic, that will be reflected in patient interactions, and even treatment decisions. Physicians must be on guard not to allow their conflicts with management to negatively impact the quality of their clinical care.

Case 12

Mr. M was a 50-year-old man with anxiety, multiple somatic complaints, and persistent difficulty adjusting to the demands of life. Dr. C provided medications for him through CMH, where he also received concurrent psychotherapy. His condition was quite resistant to improvement, and his sessions entered a routine of patient complaint and physician hopelessness.

During a typical visit, Mr. M presented a litany of problems in his family and personal life. Dr. C found herself sharing his despair. As the time to end the appointment approached, she experienced significant relief at the thought that she was really only responsible for his medications, which had recently been adjusted and did not need to be changed. She reflected that the session would soon end and her own sense of hopelessness would soon be shelved for another few weeks. She then became aware that she was no longer listening to what he said.

As she ended the session, he asked, "Do you really care about any of this?"

Dr. C used her understanding of her limited role in the medication clinic as a defense against the hopelessness she shared with the patient. Not surprisingly, he recognized her emotional distance during the session, and responded accordingly.

WORKING WITH TRANSFERENCE AND COUNTERTRANSFERENCE DURING TREATMENT

Recognition of the impact of the patient's and the physician's assumptions, expectations, feelings, and reactions on their work together is critical, but is only the first step in effective work with these issues. Throughout the course of treatment, attention to transference and countertransference, elucidation of its impact on the treatment, and work to support its positive effects while minimizing its negative impact are essential.

Initial Evaluation

In the early phase of medication treatment, most work with transference and countertransference will be focused on expectations and assumptions about diagnosis and treatment. It is usually helpful to elicit from the patient as early as possible the purpose of the visit—not only the chief complaint, but the expectation of what will be done. In this context, the psychiatrist should explicitly state the treatment options available, even before beginning the clinical interview. Initial steps that will facilitate work with transference issues are outlined in Table 5.3.

The initial diagnosis should be presented with careful attention to the patient's reaction, and sensitivity to the meaning of the diagnosis for the patient. Often clues to what to expect will be given during the clinical interview; especially past psychiatric history and family history of psychiatric illness will suggest preexisting notions regarding diagnosis. Although it is rarely appropriate to withhold diagnostic information from patients, the decision of how much information to present, and how to frame it, must be handled with sensitivity in every initial assessment.

In general, it is preferable to emphasize the positive aspects of having a correct diagnosis. The benefits include acknowledgment of the patient's suffering, encapsulation of distress into a diagnostic category, the possibility of an accurate prediction of the course of symptoms, and the likelihood of effective treatment. Care should be taken to avoid the negative aspects of receiving a named diagnosis, including the attachment of a label to the patient, dismissal of the patient's distress, catastrophic thinking regarding the course of the disorder, or a reductionist view that the disorder occurs independently of the patient's life.

Patient education regarding the diagnosis is the single most effective step to be taken initially, and should be given in virtually every case. The patient's reaction should be monitored closely. Misunderstandings, inaccurate assumptions, and catastrophic thinking should be recognized and discussed promptly. The patient's understanding and feelings about the diagnosis should be elicited and discussed.

The patient's views, values, and preferences regarding treatment should also be explored. The positive and negative aspects of each available form of treatment should be presented as objectively as possible. As in the case of diagnosis, patient education regarding treatment should be a part of every initial evaluation. Many misconceptions, unrealistic expectations, and false assumptions can be corrected with early presentation of clear and detailed information. The patient's responses, both verbal and nonverbal, should be closely monitored. It should not be assumed that silent patients are without concerns or complaints. Affective re-

TABLE 5.3. Steps in Dealing with Transference Issues

Initial steps	• Determine patient preferences
	• State physician preferences
	• Educate the patient regarding diagnosis and treatment
	• Discuss treatment options
	• Emphasize the unique value and risks of each treatment option
	• Consider the real situation
	• Maintain a neutral stance regarding treatment choice
Follow-up steps	• Maintain open communication
	• Listen for patterns and meanings
	• Assess patient compliance
	• Assess patient response
	• Assess side effects
	• Consider the real situation
	• Review patient education
	• State recommendations and their justification clearly
	• Keep other treatment options open

sponses such as physical stiffening, reduction in spontaneous conversation, hesitation, or the appearance of concern should be noted and explored. Appropriate responses to a negative reaction from a patient include education, adjustment of the treatment plan, and discussion of historical or personal reasons for the patient's concerns.

Examination of the physician's stance in this setting is also crucial. Patients respond differently to authoritarian and nondirective approaches. Although the fundamental recommendation lying behind the statements, "You need medication," and, "One tool we haven't considered yet is medication," is the same, they represent radically different approaches to the patient. The degree of rigidity or flexibility with which the psychiatrist approaches the patient is also important to monitor. While most patients respond well to reasonable flexibility in selecting treatment, dependent or anxious patients may respond more favorably to a firmer stance. Astute clinicians observe their own patterns of behavior in these relationships, as well as their patients' responses, and make adjustments accordingly.

Case 13

Ms. D was a 33-year-old woman who presented a history consistent with a first episode of major depressive disorder. Dr. S explained the diagnosis, which Ms. D already suspected. Dr. S asked if the patient had preferences regarding treatment, such as medication versus psychotherapy, or a specific antidepressant medication. The patient stated that she had no preferences, but was willing to accept whatever treatment Dr. S recommended. Dr. S suggested a common antidepressant, BB. The patient said nothing, but visibly stiffened, and appeared distracted.

Noting the change in her demeanor, Dr. S commented, "You seem uncomfortable. Do you have a concern about this medication?"

Ms. D responded, "I have a friend who took that drug and had a terrible time. I'm surprised that you would recommend such a bad drug for me."

Dr. S struggled to minimize the defensive feelings that immediately arose.

She said, "Our purpose here is to help with your depression. Antidepressant BB works well for a lot of people, but, like all medicines, it may have some side effects. Did your friend find a different medicine that was more helpful?"

Ms. D gave the name of another common first-line antidepressant.

"That would be a fine choice, as well. Would you like to use that one?"

Dr. S adjusted her initial recommendation and started treatment with the patient's preferred medication.

Despite Ms. D's initial refusal to say so, she had strong feelings about specific antidepressants, which Dr. S noted. She quickly adjusted her treatment plan to take this into account, avoiding potential problems later in treatment.

Follow-Up Evaluation

The roles of transference and countertransference typically become more prominent as treatment progresses, and the clinician should be attuned to these issues. For this reason, session times must not become excessively brief. In general, 25- to 30-minute follow-up sessions will provide a more satisfactory course than more truncated visits. Even in a crowded clinic schedule, however, with very brief appointment times (15 to 20 minutes), a significant part of each session should be devoted to discussion of the patient's feelings, experiences, and reactions. Sessions should begin with a series of open-ended questions about the patient's condition generally, while questions to elicit specific side effects or degree of symptom improvement can be handled quickly later in the session. Most patients welcome the opportunity to talk with their physicians, even if only for a few minutes. These minutes are invaluable for the clinician as well, opening a window into the patient's life that would otherwise be inaccessible. A possible outline for follow-up sessions is given in Table 5.4.

The goals of the psychiatrist in this phase of treatment are to come to know the patient well, to observe patterns of behaving, perceiving, and responding to the world, to maintain open lines of communication, and to keep treatment options open (Dewan, 1992). Some assumptions that the patient makes about symptoms and their treatment will only become clear with the passage of time. Similarly, patterns of noncompliance, frequent complaints of side effects, descriptions of inadequate treatment response, and complaints about other aspects of the clinical service suggest issues that need to be explored. Maintenance of open communication with the patient will allow opportunities for the psychiatrist to comment on these patterns as they emerge. Specific steps to be taken in follow-up interviews are outlined in Table 5.3.

TABLE 5.4. Suggested Schedules for 15- and 30-Minute Medication Visits

Activity	30-minute session	15-minute session
Open-ended questions	15 minutes	5 minutes
Follow-up questions	5 minutes	2 minutes
Specific questions regarding treatment response	3 minutes	2 minutes
Specific questions and discussion of side effects	2 minutes	2 minutes
Discussion of treatment plan	2 minutes	2 minutes
Patient education	2 minutes	1 minute
Prescriptions	1 minute	1 minute

At this stage of treatment, a listening ear and a willingness to take a few minutes to investigate pertinent issues become critical factors in positive outcome. It is never safe to assume that all aspects of the patient's feelings about the illness, treatment, or other issues have been adequately elucidated. In general, even in a brief appointment, there is time to address these issues.

Case 14

Ms. R was a 30-year-old woman receiving treatment for depression and anxiety through an interdisciplinary mental health clinic. She was assigned to a master's-level therapist for weekly 1 hour sessions and to Dr. G, a psychiatrist, for monthly 30-minute medication visits. As was typical for the clinic, her therapist was required to write specific goals for each session, specific interventions directed toward those goals, and an evaluation of the patient's progress in each session. The patient commented to Dr. G that the therapy seemed contrived and forced. In contrast, her medication visits, though brief, were largely unstructured in format and supportive in approach. Much of the available time was spent with Dr. G simply listening to her concerns. She responded well to the first antidepressant prescribed, had few side effects, and needed little attention to her medication. "To tell you the truth," she commented, "I think these visits do me more good than the therapy."

Ms. R reflected her feelings of support within the therapeutic relationship established with Dr. G in the medication clinic. Although there may well have been other issues in the psychotherapy that led to the patient's critical assessment, it is clear that her work in the medication clinic was viewed in a most positive and beneficial light.

Medication Changes and Dose Adjustments

Just as a diagnosis has meaning for the patient, so too does treatment. This becomes especially pertinent when changes in medication or dosage are recommended. When these changes are initiated by the patient, the physician does well to listen carefully to the overt reason for the requested change, and also to consider what underlying factors might be in play. It is critical to note what emotions are expressed or implied, and what they signify.

Similarly, the psychiatrist's response to the possibility of a change in treatment must be monitored. Frustration, defensiveness, hopelessness, and anger are common. Does the medication change represent a personal failure? Is there any real expectation that the patient's symptoms will improve? Is there a pattern in the physician's selection of times for dose changes? Does every visit include some adjustment? Do adjustments occur only when the patient speaks of suicide?

In general, clear reasons for every change should be stated, as should the expected benefit of the change. Adjustments that seem less readily justified should be examined more closely.

Case 15

Mr. E was a 34-year-old man with a history of psychosis, maintained for several years on an antipsychotic medication. Although Mr. E had mentioned a low level of continuing symptoms during several clinic visits, Dr. L responded with reassurance that his response was actually quite good, and ordered no change in medication.

Dr. L was surprised to receive a telephone call from Mr. E's supervisor at work, who stated that Mr. E had deteriorated significantly over the past several weeks, often complained of psychotic symptoms at work, and had expressed frustration with the ineffectiveness of his medications.

At their next visit, Dr. L reported the telephone call to his patient. Dr. L recommended an adjustment in the dose of the antipsychotic medication. Mr. E expressed frustration and anger that his own concerns had been ignored until they were substantiated by his supervisor.

Dr. L's resistance to medication adjustment was based on his assumption that psychotic disorders do not remit entirely with treatment, and led to insufficient attention to the patient's individual situation. Mr. E's anger at not being taken seriously was well founded.

Side Effects

Medication side effects not only have immediate physical consequences, but also implications in the minds of the patient and physician. For the patient, initial fear of the medication, resistance to treatment recommendations, denial of illness, or anger at the physician, diagnosis, or treatment may be reinforced by medication side effects. The converse may also occur, in which the patient's negative countertransference to treatment may be expressed as complaints of side effects that otherwise might not be noticeable or significant.

Among the most troublesome of side effects in this regard are sexual dysfunction, weight gain, impaired cognition, and movement disorders. These are problems in their own right, but also carry important transference implications.

Sexual dysfunction often goes unreported because of patient embarrassment and an inadequately trusting relationship with the physician. Sexual function, as well as dysfunction, may carry unstated meaning for the patient, such as rigid moral implications, suggestions about one's sexual capacity or orientation, fears of aging, or implications for other types of intimacy. These can only be explored after careful groundwork has been laid for a trusting therapeutic relationship.

The most important steps to avoid these transference problems are the early establishment of free lines of patient-physician communication, effective initial patient education, and careful attention to the patient's concerns from the outset of treatment. These measures are most useful when instituted before problems occur, and are more difficult to initiate later in treatment. In the middle phase of treatment, verbal exploration of the patient's concerns and behaviors may bring to light the underlying issues, which can then be addressed directly.

Noncompliance

Numerous studies have found that up to 50% of patients are noncompliant with medications or other treatment at some point during their care. Failure of the patient to follow through with prescribed treatment after a careful initial discussion and adequate education strongly suggests transference issues (Book, 1987). Although the appropriate initial response of the psychiatrist should include further education and behavioral interventions (e.g., a pillbox), prompt exploration of psychodynamic issues is also indicated.

Perhaps the most common defensive response to medications is denial—the deletion from consciousness of unpleasant material. In this case, medication doses force the patient to confront at least once every day the reality of illness, the threat of functional loss, the need for treatment, an implication of dependency, and a sense of personal inadequacy. The patient is able to avoid facing these issues by forgetting to take the medicine.

Failure to comply with treatment may also represent a more direct expression of the patient's ambivalence about the diagnosis or treatment. Patients' commitment to treatment may be limited by their difficulty accepting a psychiatric diagnosis, unwillingness to feel dependent on the physician or medication, fear of debilitating or irreversible medication side effects, or concern over social stigma.

Anger at the diagnosis, treatment, psychiatrist, clinic, or other aspects of the patient's life is often expressed as treatment noncompliance. The anger may be overt, in which the patient will make a conscious decision not to comply with treatment, or it may be unconscious, in which the patient may act in a variety of maladaptive and destructive ways to subvert treatment. In extreme (but not rare) cases, the patient may express anger by overdosing on the very medication prescribed to address the apparent problem.

These issues will yield more readily to psychodynamic exploration than to other interventions, such as additional patient education or behavioral measures.

Case 16

Mr. N was a 27-year-old single man of conservative Christian upbringing and practice, who was referred to Dr. J's medication clinic by his minister for treatment of anxiety. He gave a 6-month history of recurrent panic attacks without agoraphobia, and was prescribed an appropriate medication for long-term treatment. At each of his return visits he rather curtly described the medication as "fine," and denied recent panic symptoms. In contrast to his verbal report, he consistently looked distressed, and acknowledged that he was functioning below his baseline at work. With careful questioning, he revealed that he had not been taking the medication, and that his panic attacks had continued unabated. He expressed ambivalence about the diagnosis, noting that the attacks only occurred intermittently, and had not been a problem through most of his life. Furthermore, he considered this a failure of his religious faith, which he felt should spare him such vicissitudes. Dr. J addressed with him the meaning of his faith and the implications of his symptoms. With Mr. N's permission, his minister, who was supportive of treatment, was also involved.

Mr. N's assumptions regarding the meaning of his diagnosis and treatment were the major issues in his care. Dr. J's ability to address these issues was crucial to the patient's successful treatment.

Treatment-Refractory Patients

Treatment failure arouses significant feelings in both the patient and the psychiatrist. Transference feelings may include anger, hopelessness, frustration, or suspicion. Although few positive transference reactions are likely to arise in such cases, more narcissistic patients may feel that failure of conventional treatment confirms their sense of being unique or special. In fact, initial treatment failure may open the opportunity to broaden the treatment and may allow development of a stronger treatment alliance with a psychiatrist who remains committed to the patient's welfare despite the extra effort required.

Countertransference feelings to treatment failure may include anger, guilt, defensiveness, hopelessness, or therapeutic nihilism. There is a tendency to drift toward the extremes of optimistic continuation of ever-more obscure medication combinations or acceptance of the patient's condition as untreatable. The more reasonable approach—to have an outline of rational treatment options subject to review and revision, and consultation for additional opinions—is difficult to maintain in the face of powerful feelings of failure and inadequacy. Ironically, the most effective step the psychiatrist can take at this point is consultation, if only to confirm that the problem is refractory symptoms, not incorrect diagnosis, overlooked features, or inadequacy of treatment.

An additional concern with treatment-refractory patients is the possibility that psychodynamic issues may contribute to treatment failure. This issue must be approached with great care and sensitivity to avoid the implication that the patient is to blame for the lack of response. In the context of transference, treatment response may carry negative implications for the patient, suggesting that the precipitating problems were not as severe as imagined, that less depression or anger may absolve past offenders in the patient's life, or that it may be necessary to take a more active role in determining one's fate. Exploration of the patient's response to treatment failure may reveal for the first time the patient's opposition to medications or other therapies in use.

Countertransference feelings may be a useful tool at this time, yielding information about the patient's affect and interpersonal style that were not obvious earlier. Subtle character pathology may be detected for the first time in this setting, as may other dynamic issues related to early family experiences, patterns of relationship, or self-concept. Sensitivity to the psychiatrist's affective responses to the patient may be helpful in detection of these issues.

Case 17

Mr. U was a 34-year-old man who presented himself to Dr. K's medication clinic for treatment of depression and angry outbursts. His history included a lifetime pattern of suspiciousness and avoidance of interpersonal relationships. His depression was mainly related to his perception that others harbored malice toward him, and his frustration at not being able to maintain employment or relationships under those circumstances. He stated that he was not interested in exploratory psychotherapy, but just wanted something to reduce his distress at the situation.

Dr. K was attentive to the paranoid traits in Mr. U's interpersonal style, and stayed within that framework for the first few months of their unsuccessful treatment, including both antidepressant and antipsychotic medications. Mr. U became increasingly angry and frustrated with treatment, but continued to attend medication reviews and report good compliance.

While discussing the case with a supervisor, Dr. K noted that her countertransference was not the fear and defensiveness she would expect in response to a paranoid, angry patient, but rather boredom and a significant absence of affective connection. Prior to the next session, she reviewed Mr. U's initial history, and noted for the first time that there were significant avoidant traits that she had not noticed previously. During their next session, Dr. K asked less about Mr. U's suspiciousness of people, and more about his frustrated longing for connection. Although they had only a few minutes to discuss the issue, Mr. U acknowledged that this was a key issue in his distress. Over the next few visits, Dr. K reframed the questions she used to evaluate the effectiveness of medication, and made treatment decisions based on this new insight, with good results.

Mr. U's failure to respond to treatment was driven, in part, by an incomplete diagnostic formulation. Dr. K's attention to countertransference issues was critical to correct the problem.

CONCLUSION

As in psychotherapy, transference and countertransference feelings have a prominent role in the medication clinic. Positive transference toward the psychiatrist, diagnosis, medications, and clinic setting will help maintain a strong treatment alliance that will encourage compliance, perseverance, and good treatment outcome. Negative transference will undermine these goals. Similarly, the psychiatrist's countertransference feelings have a significant impact on the course of treatment, and may be a useful tool during the course of therapy.

The astute psychiatrist will be attentive to these issues in the medication clinic. With the many competing demands on the physician's time in the clinic, it becomes more, not less, important to be attuned to psychodynamic issues in play during the course of medication treatment. Awareness and use of transference and countertransference feelings will enhance the psychiatrist-patient relationship, improve patient compliance, and positively affect treatment outcome.

CHAPTER SIX

Managing Split Treatment

Case 1

Mr. A, a 20-year-old male university student, was referred to one of us by his psychotherapist for what the therapist thought were a mixture of depressive symptoms and some anxiety symptoms. The patient had a long history of awkward interpersonal relationships as well as inconsistency in his schoolwork. He avoided most intimate relationships and also had a history of what appeared to be moderate alcohol abuse. However, when he was seen by the psychiatrist who was to do the prescribing, it became clear that he was much more anxious than depressed. His depression seemed to be secondary to the exhaustion he experienced during periods when his anxiety was running exceptionally high. The psychiatrist suggested an SSRI to help the anxiety and also said that he would call the psychotherapist about his recommendation. The psychotherapist was at first reluctant to go along with the recommendation for medication because he feared that the fluoxetine would reduce the patient's anxiety to such a degree that the patient might not work as effectively in psychotherapy. The psychiatrist disagreed, saying that he felt the medications would permit a reduction of anxiety to a degree that would make the therapy more productive. The therapist and psychiatrist agreed to monitor the situation by frequent telephone contacts between them. This would allow them to attend to the therapist's fears; help the patient to undergo an adequate trial of the medication; and eliminate any possibility the patient would get caught in between the therapist and the psychiatrist. Mr. A responded well to the SSRI, and his anxiety was significantly reduced to the extent he could not only concentrate on his schoolwork but also maintain a steadier posture in his interpersonal relationships. It is difficult to determine whether it was the medication alone that helped with this latter problem, or whether the medication reduced his anxiety to such a degree that he could work on and discuss more productively in therapy his fears and anxiety about interpersonal situations. After about a year had passed since the initiation of the medications, Mr. A decided that he no longer wanted therapy and wanted just to be on medications and to meet with the psychiatrist about once every three months. He did feel that the psychotherapy had been helpful. In discussions with the therapist it was clear that he felt that Mr. A was prematurely terminating the treatment, and that the medications were the reason for the early termination. It was difficult for the therapist to understand that whatever the reason for the improvement and/or the termination, Mr. A was now substantially better than when he had first initiated treatment.

Frequently, treatment is delivered under conditions of split treatment. By split treatment we mean that one person is managing the medications and another is managing other aspects of the treatment. The most common version is a psychotherapist who conducts the nonmedical part of the therapy and a psychiatrist or primary care physician who manages the medications. Yet there are other combinations: Treatment can be split between a psychiatrist managing the psychotropic medication and an internist managing other medical problems, for example.

Split treatment demands cooperation and communication among the various people providing the treatment, the people we call the treaters. At the outset, this communication among treaters may appear to be more time consuming than it is worth. Yet, in the long run it helps avoid conceptual splits and disagreements among the members of the treatment team and helps minimize the opportunity for the patient to consciously or unconsciously take advantage of the split in treatment. The communication process involves each member of the treatment team having some knowledge of, as well as respect and appreciation for, what the other member(s) of the treatment team are doing. In addition it provides the patient with a more comprehensive, coordinated, and integrated treatment than she or he would otherwise receive.

SPLIT TREATMENT: DEFINITIONS AND SCENARIOS

Split treatment is far from an unusual situation, and it appears that the psychiatrist (or primary care physician) in the role of "medication backup" person is becoming increasingly common (Riba & Balon, 1999). In addition, there are other circumstances where medication backup occurs as well, most commonly when another physician is providing the medical care. For example, a primary care physician may feel too unfamiliar with psychotropic medications to prescribe them effectively and request a referral to a psychopharmacologist. Or the primary care physician may have tried a number of psychiatric medications without success and might need a backup. Or the patient has a chronic, serious medical condition and the specialist physician dealing with that particular problem lacks familiarity with psychotropic medications or just doesn't want to deal with mental health issues or treatment. In a few instances, the psychiatrist is asked to provide periodic consultations to the prescribing primary care physician while the primary care physician manages the psychotropic medications day-to-day. But whatever the circumstance, the psychiatrist is the prescribing physician while the patient is involved in some psychological/behavioral/medical treatment with someone else, and there is a need for communication between the psychiatrist and the other person providing care.

Case 2

Ms. B is a 50-year-old married woman who is being treated by her primary care physician (PCP) for hypothyroidism, which has been stable for years. Ms. B began to experience signs and symptoms of major depression, and her PCP called Dr. B, a psychiatrist, to consult on Ms. B. In the initial phone conversation, the PCP who knew Dr. B, said that while she didn't usually have any difficulty prescribing psychiatric medications on her own, she was concerned about the mixture of hypothyroidism and depression. After some discussion on the phone, including a discussion of the interplay between depression and hypothyroidism, it was agreed that Dr. B would evaluate, initiate, and stabilize the patient on antidepressant medications. After the patient was stabilized, the PCP would take over the prescribing of, and following the patient on, the psychotropic medication.

The above example can appear in many different variations. The primary care physician might want the psychiatrist to see the patient only once in order to consult and make recommendations and perhaps point out clinical signs or symptoms that need to be watched for, or might want the patient to remain with the psychiatrist even after the patient has been stabilized. Whatever the eventual long-term arrangement, communication not only at the outset but throughout the joint treatment is essential.

COMMUNICATION BETWEEN PROVIDERS DURING SPLIT TREATMENT

There are at least two types of communications that, under ideal circumstances, should take place when treatment is split. The first has to do with the straightforward issue of keeping the collaborating clinician informed with data. The second has to do with understanding and appreciating the role of the treating professional.

Keeping Treaters Informed

Issues of keeping other treaters informed seems at first glance to be quite straightforward and should present no difficulty. And yet it often does. Physicians are not known, in general, to go very far out of their way to communicate with other physicians or other nonphysician professionals. It is also not uncommon for physicians to believe that their medical degree gives them the authority over PhDs or MSWs to be in charge of the case. There are legal implications as well. In most cases, if there is litigation around a treatment, the physician is often viewed as the person in charge (or certainly the plaintiff tries to get the judge or the jury to believe that the physician is really in charge, and if the physician was not in charge of as well as familiar with all aspects of the treatment, then he was being derelict in his duty). Thus some physicians argue that since they will be liable no matter what the actual relationship between treaters really is, in truth they *are* in charge and there is little need to communicate. Of course, given the fact that liability is often shared among treaters, then good communication and knowledge and agreement around what the other person is doing is essential not only for good patient care, but to provide evidence that the treatment was well-thought, collaborative, and integrative. Keeping each other informed, and not getting split off or isolated, or not allowing one aspect of the treatment to become split off or isolated, is helpful to both good patient care as well as to avoiding disagreements or difficulties that can lead to troublesome medical or legal situations.

What are typical situations that arise? Say the primary care physician is unaware of what medications a patient is taking. He might end up prescribing medications that are metabolized by the P450 cytochrome system while the patient is taking fluoxetine (Tanaka & Hisawa, 1999). Or take the cardiologist who is unaware of the fact that a patient is taking a monoamine oxidase inhibitor; an even more serious problem could occur if the cardiologist prescribed a narcotic (Noorily et al., 1997). Simple sharing of basic information as to what a patient's pharmacologic regimen is, or how it has been modified recently, can be life-and-death information.

Another area of concern has to do with the misinterpretation of side effects. If you are the psychotherapist of a patient you see weekly, and unbeknownst to you, the psychiatrist has changed the patient's medications, you might interpret the patient's newly presented irritability and forgetfulness incorrectly. On the other side of the ledger, it would be important for the prescribing psychiatrist to know that the patient had just recalled an exceedingly traumatic childhood memory in the last therapy session prior to the patient's suddenly calling the prescribing psychiatrist to tell her that everything is falling apart, that he cannot sleep, that he is fearful and paranoid, particularly at night, and that he cannot keep it together and feels dissociated and suicidal. (Of course, as discussed earlier in this book, the psychopharmacologist should not simply prescribe or change medications without knowing what is going on in many aspects of the patient's life; and in this instance, therapy is one very important aspect. Nonetheless, even a thorough, eagerly inquiring psychopharmacologist cannot make up for the usefulness of frank open communication and exchange of information between or among those people involved in the treatment of the patient.)

Certainly, initial communication between the therapist providing the ongoing psychotherapy and the psychiatrist who is to provide the ongoing medication management is crucial, and there should always be some sort of conversation between the two providers before "joint" care is to be initiated. However, no matter how extensive this initial conversation might be, this does not excuse the psychiatrist-psychopharmacologist from doing a thorough evaluation himself or herself. An initial evaluation interview must be conducted, and as stated in Chapter 3, this cannot be accomplished in 15 minutes, and it should not be simply a symptom-based,

"Let's see if this particular symptom is there"-driven interview. Rather, the psychopharmacologist needs to establish himself or herself as a person who is interested in all aspects of the patient's life and is willing to listen to the patient's feelings and complaints even if the psychiatrist's primary role will "merely" be medication maintenance. Certainly if the patient repeatedly begins to bring in material to the psychopharmacologist that ought to be brought into the psychotherapy, this issue should be brought up and discussed, not only between the patient and the psychopharmacologist, but between the psychopharmacologist and the psychotherapist as well.

Two additional points need to be made about conducting one's own thorough initial interview. We have found it much easier to remember details about a patient's life and to have a fuller appreciation of those details and life issues when we have heard them firsthand from the patient. It is not quite the same, and it lacks richness and depth, if the information is gathered just by reading the chart or by talking with someone else about the treatment. We organize material best when we organize it ourselves, and when we ask the questions that we need to ask when we need to ask them in the interview. A second reason, discussed in more detail later, is that the referral to a psychopharmacologist by a psychotherapist provides an opportunity for consultation by another mental health professional, and without a thorough, firsthand evaluation by the psychopharmacologist, then this opportunity for genuine consultation is essentially lost.

Different understandings of observable phenomena take place when a person has different amounts of data available to him. We may want to assume that there is little need for communication between treaters because patients should be able to communicate these differences by themselves to the other people involved in their treatment. However, if the patient perceives or believes the treater does not want to listen (see Chapter 1); or if the patient had been or felt he had been rebuffed by the treater in the past; or if the patient is, in some fundamental way, passive and nonassertive; or if the patient suffers from the side effects of the medications or from increased dissociative defenses that have risen up since the remembering of the trauma, then the patient may not be able to think clearly or express himself in a reasonably articulate manner, or assert himself sufficiently to make himself heard by a busy noninterested physician. In addition, patients have different relationships with their treaters (see Chapter 5) and may be more readily able to talk to their psychotherapist than their prescribing physician. Or they may invest more authority in the prescribing physician and believe that the therapist is misguided. This patient cannot be expected to communicate readily the information needed by the other treater and the end result is a lack of communication, a fragmented case, and often failed treatment.

Case 3

Ms. C, a 55-year-old married woman was being seen by Dr. C for medication management. She was also in treatment with Ms. MSW. Because of Dr. C's schedule, he often did not return phone calls until 9 or 9:30 in the evening. Ms. C spoke with Ms. MSW about how uncomfortable she felt when Dr. C called her somewhat late in the evening at home. It felt like a date to her, and it made her uncomfortable. Ms. MSW urged Ms. C to address the issue with Dr. C, which she did and both agreed that he would not call her after 6 P.M.

One simple way to communicate among various treaters is electronically, either by facsimile (fax) or electronic mail (e-mail). Of course, if either of these types of communication is utilized, then the first thing is that each treater should have permission from the patient to speak with the other treater. If there is to be electronic communication between the treaters, then there should be a consent signed by the patient for this particular form of communication, and the patient should be aware of, and it should be stated on the consent form, that these forms of communication may not be as "secure" and confidential as other forms of communication (Kane & Sands, 1998). The great benefit of these forms of communications is the fact that they are fast, efficient, and cost-effective. If no discussion but just basic information needs to be exchanged, then these electronic forms are most useful. But if a dialogue needs to take place, then a phone call or other means of communication, where there can be give-and-take or questions and answers between the participants, needs to be employed. Also, using electronic forms of communication is only effective if both people involved in the treatment regularly connect up with their e-mail. If one of them checks e-mail only every weekend, then this should be known and the need to easily convey information must be balanced by the urgency behind the need for communication.

How often should treaters communicate? If a treatment is well established, long periods of time can go by without communication among the various treaters. The key issue is to make sure you communicate when a significant change occurs in any aspect of the treatment. These can fall into different categories, including the patient's presentation, the medication regimen; the patient's medical status, and the type of psychotherapeutic style/method used.

Respecting the Role of the Other Treaters

The second issue of communication has to do with understanding, appreciating, and respecting what the other person is providing in the treatment. The emphasis here is not whether each respects the other as a person or even as a physician (or therapist), but rather whether each provider respects what the other is doing in the treatment. In the most ideal situation, the prescriber and the therapist know each other and perhaps even work in the same clinic. If not, then at least each should know something about the other's practice, practice standards, practice behaviors, and practice beliefs.

Unfortunately, in this era of managed care, psychiatrists are often expected to write prescriptions for a whole group of nonmedical therapists, many of whom the psychiatrist knows little about. It needs to be pointed out that this arrangement is potentially very dangerous from both a clinical perspective as well as a legal one. This fact of life makes it critical for psychiatrists in this situation to have some understanding of the practice of each nonmedical therapist with whom the psychiatrist is in a split-treatment situation and is providing medication backup. (While this seems to be enormously time-consuming, it is certainly less time-consuming than finding out about the unusual practice behaviors of the other treater in a court of law.)

What's required for the psychopharmacologist to know? All psychiatrists are not experts in psychosocial interventions, but all should have an appreciation for and some fundamental understanding of the psychological issues involved in the case. This will give you the ability to monitor the degree to which these issues are prevalent or are played out in your contacts with the patient around medication issues. Further the psychiatrist ought to clearly know how contacts around medication issues will take place. Will the patient call directly? Will there be a discussion with the psychotherapist before the phone call to the psychopharmacologist? In addition, the prescribing psychiatrist needs to make clear and discuss with the therapist his or her beliefs in the efficacy or the lack of usefulness of psychotherapy in the particular disorder as well as for the particular patient under consideration. Psychotherapy of a patient in any diagnostic category cannot proceed constructively if the prescriber working with the same patient does not believe that psychotherapy is a useful undertaking.

Other issues need to be clarified as well, which we will refer to as boundary and maintenance issues. Should between-session phone calls be permitted in the pharmacologic treatment if they are not permitted or are frowned upon as part of the psychotherapy treatment? If one of the treaters usually charges for phone calls and one does not, should this difference continue or should one of the treaters modify policy in this instance? In what quantities will the pills be prescribed (especially if the patient is depressed or has a propensity for suicidal ideation or parasuicidal behavior), and what course should the therapist take if there is a sudden increase in the suicidality of the patient? Should the psychopharmacologist be contacted immediately? When the patient requests a change or an increase in dosage, will the prescriber contact the therapist beforehand to discuss what might be going on in the psychotherapy at that particular time or will the prescriber be on his or her own to make the decision based upon the clinical signs and symptoms? Does the therapist wish to be notified with each medication change, including changing the dosing of medications already being prescribed? How frequently will discussion between the prescriber and the therapist take place? What issues that come up with the prescriber should be directed back to the therapist, and will the prescriber notify the therapist that issues have come up in the "medication meetings" and that the patient has been urged to direct them back to the therapist and into the psychotherapy?

Case 4

Ms. D, a 35-year-old female receptionist, received low-dose neuroleptic medication prescribed by a psychiatrist while in therapy with a clinical psychologist. She had a long history of difficulty in interpersonal relationships that was complicated by intermittent paranoia. When these interpersonal difficulties became particularly severe, she would cut herself. Periodically she would feel that the therapy was failing, that her therapist was sadistic and deliberately trying to drive her crazy, and that she could no longer continue with the therapist. She wished to switch all her treatment to the prescriber, a person whom she knew also practiced long-term multiple-time-a-week psychotherapy. She, in her tendency to use the defense of splitting as well as in her tendency to idealize people, felt the prescriber was much more accessible, less angry, and less rigid than her therapist. After discussion between themselves, the therapist and the prescriber agreed to allow the patient to phone or to see the prescriber for short sessions during these crises; the patient also knew that if necessary, the prescriber would discuss their sessions with the therapist. The prescriber's general and usually unwavering stance was that he expected the patient, herself, to bring the issues discussed between them back to the therapist. The prescriber maintained the position that many of the patient's feelings about the therapist and about her treatment with the therapist were issues that needed to be worked out with her psychotherapist, and he emphasized his reluctance to try to medicate away these particular feelings. Information the prescriber had gotten from his initial long interview with her as well as from periodic discussions with her therapist allowed him to stress that he thought that her feelings about her therapist were very similar to the feelings that periodically plagued many of her interpersonal relationships, and these feelings needed to be worked out and understood in her therapy with her therapist. The prescriber emphasized that saying the feelings to him was not the same as saying them to her psychotherapist. The prescriber reiterated that he was always willing to reconsider his decision about not making a change in medication at any particular time, but he wanted the patient to go back and continue to meet as scheduled with her therapist for at least another month. If after that time things had not improved, he would then seriously consider a medication adjustment after a discussion between himself and her psychotherapist. Usually, she would go back to the therapist, the month would pass, and the "need" to change the medication would pass as well.

From our point of view, it makes sense to develop a formal contract that clearly delineates the respective roles of each treater as well as the expected frequency and range of, or limitations on, their communication (Appelbaum, 1991; Chiles et al., 1991). This may be especially useful when there is an ongoing professional relationship and understanding between the therapist and the prescriber, and when the two people share responsibility for a number of patients.

In a similar manner, the psychotherapist needs to have respect for the prescriber and for the intervention of psychopharmacology as well. (Certainly that is not the situation in the case vignette presented at the beginning of this chapter.) While nonmedical therapists don't need to be experts in the use of psychotropic drugs, the therapist should be aware of the specificity and indications, some of the major side effects, and the limitations of the specific psychopharmacologic treatment. Nonetheless, it will be very difficult to "successfully" prescribe medications to a patient if the patient's therapist believes there is no role for medications in treatment. This situation is made more difficult if the patient is very attached to the therapist, or if the therapist feels forced by the patient's family or the supervisor or clinic director to consider medications when he or she is dead set against them. The therapist may harbor these negative ideas for many reasons and it is good to be aware of the range of reaction. Perhaps the therapist believes medications are useless; or maybe that they are a sign of weakness; or an indication of the failure of the psychotherapy; or a loss of faith in God or other similar belief.

While therapists don't need to be experts in psychopharmacology, they must have some rudimentary knowledge of both the expected therapeutic as well as the possible side effects of specific psychotropic medications or of specific classes of psychotropic medications. The therapist needs to know how the medication can affect, both positively and negatively, the presentation of the patient in the therapist's office. Working knowledge of some of the beneficial and side effects of the medication will provide the therapist with some appreciation of what might be subjective versus what might be objective in the patient's experience in taking the medication. For example, some patients may get extraordinarily attached to a specific medication even though it appears to have little therapeutic effect; other patients may find the very idea of taking medications humiliating and shameful. The psychopharmacologist needs to appreciate these responses from the patient taking the medication even though these reactions are not listed in the *Physicians' Desk Reference.* In addition, patients with personality disorders or patients who appear to be quite regressed may be quite fixed at the transitional object level of functioning, and these particular types of patients may be particularly prone to employing medications as transitional objects (Winnicott, 1953). The therapist or prescriber who fails to fully appreciate the patient's psychological attachment to the medication may wonder why the patient is unwilling to change medications especially if the patient has repeatedly complained about the medications and/or if there had been little clear evidence that the medications had been effective. On the other hand, the therapist or prescriber who fails to fully appreciate the patient's disappointment in or rejection of the medications on psychological or symbolic grounds will continue to keep trying newer and newer and perhaps more dangerous combinations of medications (combinations that can almost be guaranteed to cause myriad side effects) rather than addressing the issue in the psychiatrist's office or discussing and trying to solve the issue with the psychotherapist (Main, 1957).

Information then needs to flow freely between prescriber and therapist, and the patient needs to be aware of this arrangement at the outset of treatment. It is probably a recipe for failure if the patient wishes to put limits on what information can be exchanged between therapist and prescriber; the patient needs to trust, even though it may be very difficult for her or him to do so, that the therapist and prescriber will use discretion as to what information is and is not shared. This understanding needs to be formalized at the beginning of treatment with the patient signing a release that will permit this free exchange of information, and the consent should be explicit as to which forms of communication will be used in the exchange of information. Further, whenever a conversation between the two treaters takes place, the patient needs to be informed. Otherwise one of the treaters may begin to say something about an event or reaction that the patient knows she has only told the other treater. Healthier patients might be able at this point to inquire as to where the treater got the information. More severely ill patients may become delusional or frankly paranoid or may invest the treater with magical powers or believe that the treater can read their mind which can then lead to all sorts of complicating situations and distorted beliefs and relationships in the treatment situation. A simple statement such as "I want you to know that I talked with your therapist last Thursday" can avoid much of this.

In addition, it is helpful if both the therapist and the prescriber are attuned to what the initiation of medication means to each of them in the treatment. It may be easier for both treaters to agree on the need for medication when there is a clear Axis I disorder, but when there are predominant Axis II traits or a prominent Axis II diagnosis present, then agreement may not be achieved so readily between the two providers. Often treaters may disagree on whether or not the patient actually has an Axis II disorder. Further, some therapists or psychopharmacologists, may believe that there is no role whatsoever for medications in the treatment of these types of patients. Others, particularly psychopharmacologists, may believe that there are really no Axis II disorders at all, but rather that all Axis II disorders are really a *forme fruste* of an Axis I disorder, and they then need to be treated vigorously with psychopharmacologic agents.

Certainly, these situations can become extraordinarily complex especially when dealing with patients who are renowned for seeing things in black or white, good or bad. These issues with respect to personality disorders are too complex to go into at this point, but they are elaborated upon elsewhere (Silk, 1999).

MANAGING REALISTIC AND UNREALISTIC EXPECTATIONS

It is not unusual for expectations on the part of all the people involved in a treatment to become unrealistic, especially if the patient appears not to be responding to the treatment. Without accurate knowledge about the effectiveness of medications and psychotherapy, clinicians' and patients' expectations are likely to become unrealistic. These expectations need to be clarified at the beginning of the treatment, especially between the two providers. If not, then a situation could evolve into one wherein each individual becomes disappointed and/or angry at the other people's involvement, investment, and capability. Such circumstances can readily lead to a failure of the combined treatment even if each part of the treatment appears to be progressing well in its own right. The final result could be the patient retreating into primarily an all-psychotherapy or an all-medication treatment, and the patient will be deprived of the possible synergistic benefits of an integrated approach to the treatment.

Case 5

Mr. E was a 25-year-old student who was admitted because of severe suicidal ideation and depression. When he came to the unit, he said that his outpatient psychotherapist wanted him put on medications and that the medications would "cure" his suicidality. While we, on the inpatient unit, thought at first that this was just grandiosity and an unrealistic expectation from a man with a severe narcissistic character disorder, it became clear that the outpatient therapist felt the same way, that is, that we could "cure" him. On further discussion with the outpatient therapist, it was clear that the therapist thought the patient was "just" depressed, and the therapist had no idea or appreciation of the patient's narcissism. We decided to ask the outpatient therapist to come to a meeting one-on-one with the attending so that there could be an open discussion with the therapist about our diagnostic, and thus prognostic, impressions of the patient without there being a public display of what we thought were some of the outpatient therapist's diagnostic shortcomings. We also thought the discussion would be a difficult-enough one that a conversation by phone would not suffice.

Alternatively, the inpatient unit can provide consultation of a different sort. In the vignette in Case 6, the inpatient staff helped a therapist work through issues that had become very difficult for him and were inhibiting his effectiveness in the outpatient treatment.

Case 6

Mr. F was a 25-year-old student who was admitted because of severe suicidal ideation and depression. When he came to the unit, he said that his outpatient psychotherapist wanted him put on medications and that the medications would "cure" his suicidality. While we, on the inpatient unit, thought at first that this was just grandiosity and an unrealistic expectation from a man with a complicated character disorder, it became clear that the outpatient therapist felt the same way, that is, that we could "cure" him. On further discussion with the outpatient therapist, it was clear that the therapist was overwhelmed by the case, wanted to get rid of the patient, and felt that nothing short of a pharmacological miracle cure could preserve the treatment and could prevent the patient from ultimately committing suicide. The therapist was invited to the unit to discuss his frustrations and fears with the senior attending, and the therapist, and in turn the patient, were each able to readjust their expectations. In fact, the unrealistic expectations (and concomitant frustrations that followed from the unrealistic expectations) were feeding off each other. The more each felt frustrated with the treatment, the more each spent time fantasizing about the "perfect cure" that must lie out there somewhere.

As Case 6 shows, everyone involved in the treatment needs to have an appreciation of the perceived efficacy as well as limitations of each of the interventions. This includes the patient as well, and may include spouses, other family members, roommates, bosses, and so forth (if permission is granted and the patient agrees to discussions with these other people). In addition, it is helpful to be able to know whether the therapist you are working with is able to tolerate treatment situations where progress is often very slow, punctuated by periods of improvement and regression, and where the long-range prognosis is often guarded but not necessarily negative. While this does not occur in every case, certainly in cases dealing with chronic affective disorders and personality disorders this ability to tolerate very slow progress is necessary; otherwise expectations are misaligned, and in one's mind there will be a tendency to blame the other treater for the slowness of the progress.

To reiterate, the ideal situation would be one where there is an ongoing dialogue and an ongoing professional understanding between the therapist and the prescriber, and where they share responsibility for a number of patients (Smith, 1989). Communication can become freer between them. The prescriber should experience no hesitation in asking the therapist why he or she wants medications considered at this time. Further questions to be asked include: Where is the impetus for medications coming from? Does the therapist think the medication will affect/change the therapeutic relationship? In turn, the prescriber should be able to let the therapist know if the prescriber feels that the therapist's expectations or wishes for the range or specificity of the effectiveness of the medication are unrealistic, and the prescriber should feel comfortable in describing what might, under the best of circumstances, be considered a reasonable response to the medications. Again, mutual respect and regular contact contributes to a freer exchange of ideas, thus keeping communication open and useful and allowing clarification of what the medication means to both therapist and prescriber.

CHEMICAL IMBALANCE VERSUS AN INTEGRATED CONCEPT OF MENTAL ILLNESS

Certainly mutual cooperation between therapist and prescriber will be seriously eroded if the patient believes that she or he has a "chemical imbalance" that is causing all of the psychiatric difficulties, and if the psychiatrist writing the prescriptions seriously feels that that is the case. (If the psychopharmacologist actually believes that it is "only" a chemical imbalance, then the psychopharmacologist cannot truly have a respect and appreciation for what the psychotherapist is doing; and as explained above, this mutual respect and appreciation is essential to the success of combined treatment.) Increasingly, patients state that they have been told that they are suffering from a chemical imbalance, and a prescriber whose practice consists primarily of psychobiological and pharmacotherapeutic interventions may be especially prone to accept this particular version from the patient of his or her dilemma. While there is probably little dispute about the role of genes in psychiatric disorders, there is currently little hard evidence that a *specific* chemical imbalance is responsible for any specific psychiatric disorder or group of disorders. Or as Reiss et al. have said: "What is often forgotten is that although the evidence for a genetic contribution to the etiology of these [psychiatric] disorders is beyond dispute, no studies indicate that genetic effects account for all the variation between ill and not ill individuals" (1991, p. 284). No one would dispute that ultimately all feelings, cognitions, and behaviors are biochemically mediated, but that does not mean that they are not psychologically motivated. Again we can turn to Reiss and his colleagues who, when speaking about "nonshared environmental effects" and their role in the development of psychopathology, opine:

> Psychiatry has been forced into the chronically uncomfortable position of straddling biomedicine and the social sciences and seems always to hunger for relief. . . . [Yet] the data simply do not permit a conception of the future centered on a straightforward biomedical answer to the fundamental question of the pathogenesis of major disorders. Indeed, a balanced image of the future contains a growing and equal partnership of the social sciences and molecular biology. (p. 290)

Certainly, the best approach would appear to be one that avoids convincing oneself or the patient that it is either psychological motivation or chemical mediation *alone* that is the root of the difficulties. A reasonable stance would seem to be one that considers both biology and psychology rather than one that tries to finally decide which of the two is paramount if not totally dominant. If both prescriber and therapist subscribe to this complex psychological/biological interplay (a biopsychosocial model), not only in their practice but in their belief system as well, then it will be easier for the patient to accept that uncertainty, ambivalence, limitation, and cooperation are part of successful everyday existence.

In either instance, if the psychotherapist believes that there is really no role for medications, or if the psychopharmacologist believes everything can be made better if only the right combination of medications is found, the coming together and modification of these two points of view and the respect of each for what the other is doing is crucial for the welfare of the patient. One way to get around these conceptual differences may be to consider the initial referral to the other person as a form of consultation; one needs not immediately accept or reject the ultimate findings of the referral/consultation, but the occurrence provides an opportunity for input from someone with a different point of view.

Case 7

Ms. G is a 22-year-old single woman with a long history of self-mutilative behavior, conflicts with her family, and substance abuse. She had been treated psychotherapeutically for what was thought to be a personality disorder, and because of her persistent suicidality and dislike of medications, she had never been treated pharmacologically. The psychopharmacologist wondered whether she might perhaps have social phobia, and perhaps her alcohol use was an attempt at self-medication of her anxiety in social situations. A recent suicide attempt had most probably been precipitated by her anxiety over an assignment to make a half-hour presentation to her class. She was referred to the anxiety disorders program for further consultation, and was treated with both monoamine oxidase inhibitors and behavioral therapy. Her substance abuse stopped, and she experienced a significant decrease in her suicidal ideation. She was no longer viewed as a personality-disordered patient, and the psychotherapist was pleased with the dramatic change that had occurred in his patient.

TRANSFERENCE AND COUNTERTRANSFERENCE IN SPLIT TREATMENT

The psychopharmacologist needs to remember that patients have strong feelings about and reactions toward healthcare providers in general, and intense transferential feelings may occur even in a therapy that is strictly psychopharmacological. Whenever medication is introduced into any therapy, it has repercussions on the transference in the psychotherapy part of the treatment. Have I gotten worse? Is the therapist about to abandon me and shift me over to the psychopharmacologist full time? Some patients present particular challenges. For example, some patients with character disorders have such intense, tenacious transferential feelings that they take on a reality of their own. In these cases, both treaters must be exceedingly careful when introducing medication as the entire treatment can easily self-destruct. Also bear in mind that some patients may not express their disappointment in the psychotherapist for the referral to the psychopharmacologist but rather may reserve the complicated reactions for the psychopharmacologist. Thus psychopharmacologists are far from immune to transferential (and in turn countertransferential), reactions.

Finally, if the psychopharmacologist is dealing with a particularly difficult or recalcitrant patient or condition, then there is a strong tendency for countertransferential reactions to these patients as well. Our own anger and rage at them (and at their unconscious anger and sadism) may lead us to want to abandon the treatment, to turn it over to the other provider, or to seize it all ourselves and finally get it under (our own) control. The best way to handle these feelings is not to isolate oneself or withdraw from the other provider but rather to share frustrations about the treatment with the other provider. More often than not, we will find that the other provider, rather than becoming critical or negative toward us or toward our aspect of the treatment, will admit that he or she was feeling similarly. This sharing of frustration can relieve tension in each provider as well as between the providers. Moreover, their open discussion about the case can lead to creative conceptualizations.

> One of us has the opportunity to consult to medical services on the issue of the "difficult patient." At the beginning of the presentation, the presenter frequently queries the medical audience as to what they think defines the difficult patient. The replies often take the form of: "The patient wants more time [medication, attention] than I or my clinic can provide"; "The patient is not getting better no matter what I try, and she is getting increasingly angry with me"; "I don't think the patient has anything serious, yet he is always in the office with some sort of complaint." The presenter acknowledges that these are probably all good reasons why the patient is viewed as difficult, but wonders if there isn't one overriding thought that clearly defines and separates the difficult patient from all others. It is the thought that the provider has that he or she would like to kill, or if not kill, then do some serious bodily harm to the patient. The audience then usually laughs, and the conference can then proceed to an open and realistic discussion of how one deals with one's own sadistic impulses toward patients who do not behave or do not get better in the way(s) we would like them to.

CONCLUSION

"In contemporary treatment situations that include a patient, a therapist, a pharmacotherapist, and a pill, the transference issues can become more complex than the landing patterns of airplanes at an overcrowded airport" (Smith, 1989, p. 80). In order to prevent the whole treatment process from plunging into a nosedive, there needs to be communication and respect among all those invested in the treatment process. In addition, there needs to be realistic expectations of what each of the individuals in the treatment process, including the patient, can accomplish given the material and psychological resources at their disposal.

Communication among the various people providing the treatment is essential. In the long run, communication helps avoid conceptual splits and disagreements between the members of the treatment team and also helps minimize the chances for the patient to consciously or unconsciously take advantage of the natural division between his providers. The communication process involves each member of the treatment team having some knowledge of, as well as respect and appreciation for, what the other members of the treatment team are doing. In addition, when all members of the team are communicating freely and openly with each other, then the patient can be provided with a more comprehensive, coordinated, and integrated treatment than she or he would otherwise receive.

A few words need to be said about the role of the patient in this joint endeavor. As stated earlier, it is often quite useful to appreciate what the patient feels about the prescribing of the medication, and all parties involved in the treatment need to keep their expectations realistic. Thus it is important to have the patient take the medication in a spirit of collaboration with the therapist and the prescriber. If one or the other is aware of possible reasons for the patient's resistance to taking medications, these reasons need to be heard, tolerated, and empathically responded to by both providers. If the prescriber and the therapist are not collaborative, their division will be picked up by the patient, and may lead to compliance issues. Ultimately, cooperation as to compliance, dosage, and willingness to take the medication should be based on how the patient does or does not experience the medication as beneficial or detrimental when compared with his or her premedication baseline affective, cognitive, and interpersonal functioning. Yet if we are unwilling to listen to how the medication is unhelpful, and to discuss among ourselves the reality and importance of the issues that patients present to us concerning the medication, then we will never hear how the medication might be helpful as well. This ability to hear both sides of the issue with respect to medications applies to the psychopharmacologist as well as to the psychotherapist and is another important aspect of the psychotherapy of prescribing.

CHAPTER SEVEN

Managing Difficult Cases

There are a multitude of factors that make the doctor-patient relationship so complex and challenging. Contributions come from patients and from doctors. As noted by Dr. Metzl in Chapter 2, the level of care and culture within the system also contribute to the effectiveness of the relationship.

Until now, we have tried to set forth some basic principles and a framework for understanding this relationship—what makes it work and what leads to problems especially in the psychotherapy of prescribing medication (Adelman, 1985; Chiles et al., 1991). We have discussed such issues as listening to patients; developing the therapeutic alliance, and transference and countertransference. Within the context of these themes, such specific topics as medication compliance and managing split treatment have been addressed.

We all have difficult cases, the ones that worry us a lot; the ones they didn't teach us in residency; the ones for whom giving a prescription for an SSRI is not going to be enough because of so many psychosocial problems and issues. While we will certainly not be able to describe all of the multiple combinations of problems that can occur within the doctor-patient relationship that contribute to such clinical troubles, we will try to highlight a few major themes that seem to herald or almost predict such dilemmas—the ones that when the first sentence is out of the presenter's lips, you know there is a great potential for doctor-patient problems!

Case 1

Mrs. G is a 47-year-old second-grade teacher and mother of two teenagers. Diagnosed with breast cancer 6 years ago, she tolerated the lumpectomy, chemotherapy, and radiation without significant problems. She had no previous psychiatric history and was generally doing well until she started having back pain and a persistent cough. The now-metastatic breast cancer was overwhelming to her. She could not face losing her hair again or feeling fatigued and drained from other forms of chemotherapy or from the cancer itself. Her marriage had not been great for some years and her two teenage girls were tired of having "a sick mom" who didn't look or act like their friends' mothers. She had no close relatives living nearby and her support system consisted of several women from her church and one fellow teacher. Her oncologist referred her for psychiatric care because she was delaying making some of the diagnostic and treatment issues that her oncologist thought were in her best interest.

Mrs. G was not clear what she wanted from the psychiatrist and in fact didn't think she belonged in a psychiatrist's office at all. She was only there because her oncologist "forced" her to do so. She was angry that this was happening to her again; angry that her family was not understanding; angry at her doctors who should have known what to do to prevent this from occurring. She was not interested in talking about her feelings. Mrs. G made it understood that she would not take any mind-altering medications because she didn't want to take anything that might promote her cancer to spread even further.

How does one begin to think about forging a relationship with Mrs. G? What makes this case so difficult? What are some key principles upon which to build this partnership? What are some obstacles for both the patient and doctor as well as some opportunities? (See Table 7.1.)

SETTING UP THE PARAMETERS OF THE RELATIONSHIP

One of the obvious problems is that the patient feels forced to be seeing a psychiatrist. This is a very common occurrence with medically ill patients who are advised or strongly recommended to see a psychiatrist. Sometimes the consultation is "demanded" by the primary provider, in this case an oncologist. The patient often perceives the consultation as a "requirement," not something that might be helpful.

TABLE 7.1. Potential Obstacles in Developing a Strong Psychiatrist-Patient Relationship with the Medically Ill

---

- Patient unsure of need for psychiatric attention
- Many other types of doctors are also seeing the patient
- Other types of pressures—family; financial; time
- Competition among doctors for patient's attention
- Stigmatization regarding mental health issues
- Overlap of medical and psychiatric symptoms
- Patient is already taking a lot of medication; resistance to taking more medication (e.g., psychotropics)

The patient often gets annoyed that the primary physician is having him or her see a multitude of doctors. It is time consuming and sometimes very expensive. Often, the patient isn't told exactly why a psychiatrist's services are being requested and the patient wonders if the referring doctor thinks he or she is crazy. Sometimes, patients even view it as a form of abandonment—that the primary doctor is too busy or uninterested or that the patient is a hopeless case and is being shipped off to a "shrink." Additionally, it is often very stigmatizing for patients to see a psychiatrist—this could be based on family history; the patient's own perception of mental illness; worry and fear about what happens in a psychiatrist's office; the public perception and handling of mental problems, and so on. So, in this case, that Mrs. G feels forced to see the psychiatrist is a difficult beginning.

What to do about it? The first thing is for Mrs. G and the psychiatrist to discuss it. They need to talk about the purpose of the visit at the first session and listen for recurrence of the topic at other sessions. This may turn out to be an important issue for Mrs. G at this time in her life. Is this, for example, a projection of how she feels about herself (hopeless) and that she feels her oncologist doesn't care about her anymore? Is she just exhausted about the prospect of going for more tests and seeing more doctors? Is she worried that she is going crazy?

This discussion is an important one because it shows the patient that the psychiatrist is not threatened by her aggressiveness and her feelings. Mrs. G needs to hear, probably over and over again, that whatever or whoever got her to the psychiatrist's office, it was probably a good idea. Some psychoeducation might also be useful—about 30 to 50% of patients with breast cancer will at some point in their care warrant a significant psychiatric diagnosis (Rowland & Massie, 1998). Such education helps align the doctor with the patient and decreases the distance between the two. It will also help Mrs. G to realize that she is not the only one with recurrent breast cancer who would need the help of a psychiatrist.

Another important issue that the psychiatrist must raise at the very first session is the confidentiality of information. Since this is a medical consultation, a letter or other acknowledgment is required to go to the referring oncologist. Mrs. G and the psychiatrist have to reach an understanding, from the very beginning, about the types of information that will and will not be going back to the oncologist. Without doing this, Mrs. G may not want to divulge feelings and problems that might, in her mind, affect her oncologic care.

Regarding the psychiatrist, there are clearly powerful countertransferential feelings that might develop. Feeling sorry for such a patient, putting oneself in the shoes of this patient, worrying about Mrs. G's children as she is doing, being angry at her husband are all ways the psychiatrist might identify or relate. At the beginning, it is important for those physicians working with the medically ill to have empathy but be able to separate from the plight of patients in order to best help them and their families. Identifying those feelings early is helpful. It is important for the doctor to not start providing vignettes of his or her own family's bouts with cancer or relating the plight of other patients' clinical situations. In other words, it is important to not cross boundaries. This is a common problem for psychiatrists not familiar with treating medically ill patients.

AS THERAPY PROGRESSES

One of the dangers with this case is first siding with the oncologist and attempting to get the patient to make decisions about her care—without first listening to her. There are probably some real time pressures and concerns and a window for providing her with the diagnostic tests and care she needs. But it will be important for Mrs. G to develop a trusting relationship with the psychiatrist and for Mrs. G to see that the psychiatrist is working with the oncology team but also wants to hear her fears and worries about the tests and treatment. Often, patients are not really worried about taking the tests—they are worried about the results. And they don't worry too much about the treatment—they worry about the side effects (nausea, vomiting, diarrhea, agitation, pain). When these potential worries are addressed and recognized, and a plan of attack is discussed, most patients are able to join forces with the treatment team.

It will be important to determine how the psychiatrist is going to also work with the patient's husband and daughters. When treating the medically ill, there are multiple patients—the family is always part of the care. This should ideally come after a therapeutic alliance has developed between the doctor and patient and when there is enough trust between the two that they can set the agenda for the necessary family meetings.

Another difficult part of treating the medically ill is determining if the psychiatric symptoms are part of the illness and side effects from treatment, or related to psychological or other causes. Most of the time it is impossible to tell and so patients are treated based on the goal of symptom relief and trying to minimize adverse side effects from psychotropic medications.

An important issue to always ask of medically ill patients is the use of alternative and complementary medicinals. Patients are usually pleased to be asked and to find that you are interested in hearing their thoughts about such preparations. It leads to a lot of interesting discussion about family folklore, view of doctors, trust in the medical system, and so on. In Mrs. G's case, she was thinking about seeing an acupuncturist and a naturopathic doctor who prescribes herbs and puts patients on macrobiotic diets. Mrs. G was thinking about doing this in lieu of following up with her oncologist since she was so disappointed that the cancer had returned. She felt desperate and wanted to try something unconventional. Actually this was the major reason for Mrs. G's "indecision" about going forward with her tests and the oncologist's treatment plan.

If the psychiatrist determines that a psychotropic medication is needed, it should be done with a whole lot of discussion. Often, even if there are acute vegetative symptoms (such as disturbed sleep; anhedonia; depressed mood) with a patient who tells you up-front that she doesn't want psychotropic medications, it is better to not try to prescribe medications at the first visit. One might mention that medication might help these symptoms but that you will wait to discuss that at the second session.

In Mrs. G's case, she might be asked to call a few days after the first session but before the second session to "check in" so the psychiatrist can see how she is doing. This allows the psychiatrist to let Mrs. G know that he is thinking and caring about her and wants to hear from her; it gives Mrs. G a chance to bring up how she is feeling and provide the progression of vegetative symptoms; and helps to forge the bond on a faster pace. In Mrs. G's case, it also gives her some autonomy—she can choose to make the telephone call and not feel forced into doing so. Some physicians are using e-mail for this purpose but the telephone is a warmer, more compassionate way to touch base with patients in real time and see how they're doing.

Finally, psychiatrists who care for patients with terminal medical conditions must help patients deal with their death and dying. Psychiatrists must be comfortable helping patients understand how to draw up living wills; discuss pain control and palliative issues; and make funeral arrangements. This is usually among the most difficult but important topics of discussion that occur in this type of doctor-patient relationship.

Patients often come to their psychiatrists when the oncologist or family members want to "keep going" with treatment and the patient wants to stop. This is a critical fork in the road and is a measure of the control patients want to have over their care and their lives. Within the doctor-patient relationship, the psychiatrist must anticipate such issues and provide a safe, nonjudgmental environment for the patient to sort this out.

There are many other issues to consider when working with patients who are medically ill, but the theme that pervades is the importance of working on the relationship between doctor and patient through the multiple phases of medical and psychiatric problems.

Case 2

Mr. H was a 47-year-old single male with a history significant for past alcohol dependence, dysthymia, and borderline personality disorder. He lives alone and recently was let go from a retail job for poor attendance. He had a past history of multiple suicide attempts with overdose and a self-inflicted stabbing to his abdomen. He would often cut his arms when he felt desperate and "in pain." In all previous times, he called the emergency department for help soon after his actions. He never left a suicide note. On one occasion, he reports going on a bridge and thinking about jumping but a police car was approaching and he kept walking.

Mr. H had no close relationships or support. Even the church that had been helping him financially told him to seek other help. His family had stopped any relationship with him 20 years ago when he was drinking heavily and stealing from his parents to pay for his habit.

He was recently seen in a local emergency department for suicidal threats but was not hospitalized. He had no medical insurance and the staff did not feel he was in imminent risk of self-harm. He denied drinking alcohol again and a breathalizer confirmed this.

Mr. H said he had no gun in his house or access to guns. He did say that he had sharp knives but if he were going to kill himself, he would mostly likely jump off a bridge or tall building. He admits that he will probably kill himself soon unless something drastically changes but he doesn't know what should or could change.

The emergency department referred the patient to see Dr. H who, on careful history, reveals a man who is chronically suicidal. He has passive as well as active suicide thoughts daily. Mr. H feels alone, ashamed, worthless, hopeless, worried about supporting himself, and a failure. Almost any help Dr. H offers—partial hospital program; antidepressant medications—is turned down by Mr. H. He is worried about his finances and doesn't qualify for medical assistance programs because he was recently employed and has some assets. Dr. H sees the patient for about two months. There isn't a day that goes by that Dr. H isn't worried about getting a call that Mr. H has killed himself. Each time Mr. H leaves Dr. H's office, his suicidal thoughts persist. He agreed to try an antidepressant but it doesn't seem to be helping his mood or his suicidal thoughts. Dr. H is very worried that Mr. H will get energized enough by the antidepressant to kill himself (see Table 7.2). Mr. H doesn't harbor any desire to "take anyone else" with him.

There are many factors that make this case so complex. Dr. H fears that in spite of his best efforts, Mr. H will still kill himself. Dr. H is angry that he is being put in this difficult situation. Dr. H is perplexed that the emergency department sent him such a difficult case and wonders why they did that. Dr. H doesn't feel that he knows Mr. H even after two months. There is no bond—most of the discussion is about suicide. Dr. H has set up a contract for safety—who Mr. H should call and under what

TABLE 7.2. Mr. H's Suicide Risk Factors

- Past history of suicide attempts
- Access to weapons (guns)
- Mood disorder
- History of alcohol dependence
- Single and alone—few social supports
- Unemployed (recent loss of job)
- Financial pressures

conditions—but realizes such contracts are based on mutual trust and doesn't feel that the two of them trust each other.

SETTING UP THE PARAMETERS OF THE RELATIONSHIP

Working with chronically suicidal patients (in this case, a patient with borderline personality disorder) is one of the toughest jobs for psychiatrists or any other doctors. It invokes many primitive feelings in us, including rage, anger, wanting to protect, loss of control, and helplessness (Maltsberger, 1983; Waldinger, 1989). It is also extremely dangerous.

The first problem in some ways for Dr. H and Mr. H is trying to get the issue of suicide off the table and putting it aside so that other work can get started. With suicide always in the forefront, and with Mr. H not being clear about his intentions, Dr. H can do very little except provide a holding environment. Mr. H is allowing the issue of suicide to prevent him from getting the help he needs. The only way to move the relationship forward is for Dr. H to take the risk of helping Mr. H move the issue to the side. The risk is that Mr. H will get angry about this; feel less powerful; feel overcome by Dr. H. For Mr. H, feeling suicidal is keeping Dr. H's attention on him. Perhaps he likes that and will not want to give it up. That is the dilemma. The issue of suicide is keeping a disequilibrium in the relationship between Dr. H and Mr. H with Mr. H in the driver's seat. Any chance of having a partnership in the doctor-patient relationship is nil unless there can be some movement with the suicide issue. How to do that is the challenge.

Another major problem is that there don't seem to be any other social supports or relationships for Mr. H. It seems like he is totally dependent on Dr. H (or emergency rooms) for social interaction. Dr. H doesn't understand the etiology of Mr. H's previous work problems and is worried about encouraging him to go back to work for fear that another job termination would increase his suicidality. Dr. H is also worried about bringing up the issue of partial hospital programs or other therapists to see the patient more frequently because he doesn't want the patient to feel abandoned. The only way to deal with these issues is to discuss them with the patient. Dr. H has taken on these worries himself—joining forces with Mr. H might be dangerous but at least it will model for the patient ways to discuss issues in a collaborative manner.

AS THERAPY PROGRESSES

Dr. H is able to make some movement toward getting suicide off the table but knows that it is always lurking. An important decision that Dr. H can make is getting a second opinion. Dr. H realizes that he is very caught up with this case and wonders if someone not responsible for this patient can offer some insight. Dr. H explains to Mr. H the reason for this consultation and while Mr. H at first balks, it is the first sign that he understands the dilemma he has been putting Dr. H through. Asking for a consultation from a colleague or someone very knowledgeable in a patient with chronic suicidality is an important option to consider.

Another problem ensues as time goes on. There is a compassionate feeling that comes over Dr. H. He begins to truly feel sorry for Mr. H and starts to "let down his guard." The chronic suicidality seems to become just a familiar part of the questions that go on between the two and this is dangerous. It becomes matter-of-fact to hear that Mr. H is suicidal but since he always returns for appointments, Dr. H gets lulled into thinking that the strength of his relationship with Mr. H will keep Mr. H alive. This is unfortunate and somewhat narcissistic on the part of Dr. H—he is beginning to think that since he is such a good therapist and Mr. H comes for appointments, the risk of suicide has diminished. Far from it; Mr. H continues to feel suicidal but hasn't decided what to do. He likes Dr. H but probably not enough for it to be the sole reason that keeps him from killing himself.

The goals of therapy need to be articulated with the patient. As Mr. H moves from not keeping suicide as the central issue, other problems are going to need to replace it. What should those be? Getting back to work and starting to forge other relationships would be important goals. Dr. H needs to help Mr. H slowly work toward these goals without worrying Mr. H that he will be abandoned when these goals are reached.

Dr. H also believes that medication will be helpful for Mr. H's mood. One of the worries is that Mr. H could overdose on medication.

There are special concerns that need to be particularly discussed. Dr. H's vacations and time off are always points of concern and worry for both Dr. H and Mr. H. When Dr. H is on vacation, instead of telling Mr. H to call the covering physician if he feels suicidal, Dr. H has Mr. H see the covering physician for a regularly scheduled appointment. This seems to work well.

Another tool they use is e-mail. Mr. H is allowed to e-mail Dr. H one message a day but it cannot be related to suicidality. Mr. H understands that Dr. H may not be sitting at the computer when the message is sent but knows that probably within the 24 hours, Dr. H will read it and send him a reply. All messages go into Mr. H's file and this is understood by the patient.

Mr. H understands the limits of confidentiality of information between them. When and if Dr. H thinks Mr. H is very close to suicide, confidentiality will be broken and authorities may be called in to help the situation.

Dr. H weighs the risks and benefits of prescribing antidepressant medication and decides to treat Mr. H with an SSRI. Dr. H orders frequent drug levels on the antidepressant used. While there is not a good correlation between blood levels of serotonin reuptake inhibitors and efficacy, it is nevertheless helpful because Mr. H feels he is being closely monitored and likes that and Dr. H can have a better sense whether Mr. H is taking the medication or hoarding it.

Probably the most important issue to consider in this case is for Dr. H to keep up his vigilance. Some chronically suicidal patients will in fact carry out their suicidal ideation and intent. The risk is very great in this patient and so must be treated and managed as such. The issue of suicidality, in this case, is integral to the working through of the doctor-patient relationship (see Table 7.3).

TABLE 7.3. Ways of Dealing with Suicidal Patients

- Psychiatrist gets second opinion for patient
- Psychiatrist seeks consultation (discusses with colleague)
- Addressing and understanding the transference and countertransferential issues within the doctor-patient relationship
- Doctor understands and respects limits of what she or he can do to keep patient safe
- Hospitalization should be considered when appropriate
- Working out coverage for doctor's vacation; time away
- Vigilance

OTHER DIFFICULT ISSUES

Collaborating with Primary Care Physicians

Case 3

Mr. J, a 46-year-old married engineer, self-refers to the University Psychiatric Outpatient Clinic. His primary care physician (PCP) had prescribed paroxetine about three years earlier when Mr. J was experiencing job stressors and consequent financial pressures. Mr. J had had no previous psychiatric history and when his job stabilized, so did many of the other issues. Nevertheless, his PCP thought it a good idea for Mr. J to stay on paroxetine. Mr. J had not spoken with the PCP about seeing a psychiatrist but requested this visit to discuss the need for continued medication.

This is a difficult case. What makes it so complicated? To start, Mr. J doesn't feel that he is in a partnership with his PCP even though he has received care from the PCP for over three years. Given that Mr. J didn't tell the PCP that he was seeing a psychiatrist, what is the meaning that can be derived from this break in the doctor-patient relationship? Ostensibly, the problem is presenting as a *medication* issue in that the PCP is prescribing something and either the patient doesn't trust the doctor's judgment or doesn't like taking medications and wants someone else to discontinue it; or there are other issues at play between the patient and the doctor.

For the clinic psychiatrist, how is this situation best handled? Should the psychiatrist try to explore the issues between Mr. J and the PCP or simply focus on the signs and symptoms that Mr. J is having and determine whether paroxetine is the best agent at this time? Should the psychiatrist explore the issue of psychotherapy as an adjunct or primary form of treatment for Mr. J? Is it reasonable that the psychiatrist insists on sending a copy of the evaluation to the PCP or calling the PCP? If the psychiatrist does this, is she colluding with the problems between Mr. J and the PCP?

Interestingly, most of the antidepressant medication prescribed in the United States is by PCPs, not psychiatrists (Valenstein, 1999). More depression and anxiety symptoms are being recognized by PCPs due to increased education, clinical guidelines and pathways, and better-informed patients (Lazarus, 1995). The type of depression and anxiety seen by PCPs, however, is usually different than that seen by psychiatrists. PCPs treat patients with depression and anxiety in the context of other medical problems and usually address just the major symptoms because of time constraints and knowing that they will be seeing the patient again for a follow-up appointment. When depressive or anxiety symptoms are noted by PCPs, patients are usually prescribed a medication. Psychotherapy is not often discussed and even when patients are already in psychotherapy, the communication between mental health provider and PCP is usually not very good.

Another problem illustrated by this case is what the optimal communication should be between the psychiatrist and Mr. J's PCP. This will be decided mostly by the patient—whether or not Mr. J consents to allow the psychiatrist to contact the PCP. What if the patient does not provide consent? If the psychiatrist decides to change the medication—either increase, change, or discontinue it—the quality of care could be compromised if the PCP is not provided this information. Mr. J may say that he himself will inform the PCP of any changes—but can the psychiatrist trust that that will happen? So soon in the relationship between the psychiatrist and Mr. J there are already issues of trust!

Finally, is there liability for the psychiatrist if the information is not provided to the PCP? We know that there are many drug-drug interactions between antidepressants and other common medications that may be prescribed in the future by the PCP.

Mr. J could alternatively give consent to the psychiatrist but then the psychiatrist is acting as a middleman by letting the PCP know that there are problems in the doctor-patient relationship. Perhaps this is a useful outcome but what should the psychiatrist be advised about that communication issue?

With the increase of PCPs and other physicians prescribing psychotropic medication, there continues to be a proliferation of multiple party relationships that will make the prescribing of medication even more difficult.

Working with Nonphysician Mental Health Colleagues

At many outpatient psychiatric clinics and in private practice, the first professional to evaluate a patient is a nonphysician (psychologist, social worker, counselor, etc.). In fact, often it is a nonphysician who is making the referral for medication. It is important to note that Section 5.4 of *The Principles of Medical Ethics with Annotations Especially Applicable to Psychiatry* specifically states, ". . . the physician should not delegate to the psychologist or, in fact, to any nonmedical person any matter requiring the exercise of professional medical judgment" (American Psychiatric Association, 1995). Whether the patient is being seen for psychotherapy and is subsequently referred for a medication evaluation or the referral is made early in treatment, the patient is being given either subtly or directly some notion of the importance of medication in relieving the symptoms.

If the referral to a psychiatrist is made initially by the nonphysician therapist, then the role that medication will play in the resolution of symptoms may seem extremely important, even overvalued, to the patient.

Case 4

Mrs. K, 56 years old with two married children and no previous psychiatric history, was having difficulty sleeping at night. Her husband had been diagnosed with multiple myeloma two days earlier. Mrs. K's friend had recommended a social worker in town who saw Mrs. K. for an initial consultation and recommended at that session that she see a psychiatrist for a medication evaluation. The soonest the patient could be seen by the psychiatrist was one week. Mrs. K felt that the social worker wasn't being helpful because Mrs. K came for a specific problem and wasn't getting the help she needed. She couldn't see how she was going to wait a week and when the social worker suggested ongoing supportive psychotherapy, Mrs. K was too angry and upset to see any value in either.

The difficulty in this case illustrates how problematic it often is for non-physicians without medical training to be put in the role of having to make an evaluation of the need for medication (Woodward et al., 1993). In Mrs. K's case, the role of medication perhaps became overvalued and the curative factor in the eyes of the patient. Since the social worker was unable to prescribe the medication, Mrs. K became angry and upset and did not have quick resolution of her symptoms, as she had hoped.

Perhaps the social worker did not feel that medications were key yet wanted to be on the safe side and have a psychiatrist make that determination. Without more clinical information, it is hard to know if the referral to the psychiatrist could have waited until the bond between the social worker and patient was stronger. If the referral is made for a patient who has been in psychotherapy for some time, there are additional complications in the ways the patient understands medication:

Case 5

Dr. S, a 63-year-old gay physician, was in a 5-year-long psychotherapy with a psychologist for narcissistic personality disorder. Dr. S was beginning to feel a sense of loss of self-esteem as more junior physicians were being hired in the department and were getting more of the plum assignments. The psychologist noted the patient to have symptoms of major depression and made a referral to a psychiatrist. Dr. S felt narcissistically injured, rejected, and abandoned by the psychologist, as if the psychologist were giving up. Dr. S felt that all the work he had done with the psychologist was for naught because medication was going to "numb" him and change his feelings about himself. While Dr. S didn't like the feelings of low self-esteem, he felt that it was important to work through the issues and not have a medication try to solve the problems. After years of working in psychodynamic therapy, the patient did not view his problems as biologically driven and saw no need to receive medications.

Introducing a third person (patient–nonphysician therapist–psychiatrist) into treatment is usually difficult and brings with it some of the problems evidenced in Case 5 (American Psychiatric Association, 1980b). Further complexities include how much information the psychologist in the case of Dr. S should provide to the psychiatrist. After 5 years, the psychologist had gotten to know Dr. S quite well. Clearly, some information is appropriate to share with the psychiatrist, but what will the impact be on the relationship between the psychologist and Dr. S after this information is shared?

For the psychiatrist, it is also difficult to share treatment with a nonphysician. Issues of control, who is in charge of the patient; who has the "deep pockets" if there is a lawsuit; who is responsible for development and follow-through of a treatment plan, and so forth are all potential areas of conflict. Unless the psychiatrist works regularly with the social worker or psychologist, effective ways of communication must be worked out between the clinicians and with the patient (Gardner & Holzman, 1983).

Case 6

Ms. H is a 19-year-old first-year college student being treated for eating disorder NOS by a social worker and taking sertraline for depressive symptomatology, which was prescribed by a psychiatrist. After a visit from her parents, she became quite depressed and started voicing suicidal thoughts to her roommates. Ms. H was encouraged to call her social worker. The answering service noted that the therapist was out of town and all emergencies should go to the emergency room at the local hospital. The patient was admitted to the hospital and only close to discharge was the psychiatrist informed.

Unfortunately, this scenario happens all too often. Many clinicians do not discuss the contingencies for various patient emergencies with each other or with patients. Patients, therefore, have to make decisions as to whom to call for what purpose and mistakes are often made. Ms. H thought that the psychiatrist's role was just to prescribe medications. She thought that the psychiatrist was impersonal and only cared about the medication, not about her. These feelings were fueled by brief (20 minutes) and infrequent visits with the psychiatrist while those with the social worker were for longer times (1 hour) and weekly. To Ms. H, the social worker was nurturing and warm. In this case, whether a hospitalization could have been avoided would have been helpful to better understand.

Finally, psychiatrists are very often asked to see multiple patients for short visits, or medication checks. These patients may be followed for psychotherapy by nonphysician therapists in what we call "collaborative treatment." Regarding these therapists, the psychiatrists are often unaware of their skill level, the type of care provided, education attainment, knowledge of medication, and so on. Misunderstandings can develop regarding patient care and it may become confusing as to which clinician will take care of what problem. Some work has been written about optimal ways to communicate and learn of each other's credentials, but when clinicians are busy, there are often lapses in such issues (Appelbaum, 1991). The following is an example:

Case 7

Mrs. D, a 52-year-old single woman, had been seen by a psychiatrist for 3 months for issues related to the loss of her mother and sister to breast cancer. The psychiatrist recommended starting an antidepressant but the patient refused, saying she wanted to try to deal with her problems without drugs. Since medication wasn't being provided, she asked to be referred to a psychologist for therapy. The psychiatrist wrote down the name of a psychologist, Dr. W, who recently moved into the same professional building as the psychiatrist. Several months later, the psychiatrist read in the newspaper that Dr. W had been working without a license, after losing it in another state due to sexual misconduct with patients. The psychiatrist had not checked the psychologist's credentials when making the referral and worried what the impact would be.

DIAGNOSTIC ISSUES

There has been no literature to date to determine whether patients of certain diagnostic groupings fare better with a psychiatrist who provides both psychotherapy and medication versus receiving care in collaborative treatment (a nonphysician therapist and a psychiatrist or PCP) or receiving medication alone from a PCP.

With that said, more and more we find ourselves determining practice patterns based on factors such as patients' insurance coverage, and billing issues (in an hour, a psychiatrist can see several patients who need medication versus one patient who needs psychotherapy); and there is a continuing diminution in psychiatrists who provide psychotherapy. Physicians, in general, due to such factors as time constraints, paperwork demands, and regulatory issues, rarely get copies of patients' past discharge summaries and previous clinic visits. Such neglect of taking into account the patient's diagnostic problems and past medical and psychiatric history can make the prescribing of medication complex.

Specific Diagnostic Issue: Substance Abuse

Case 8

Mrs. J is a 61-year-old married woman who is an avid jogger and retired teacher. She recently had been treated for endometrial cancer and had a good prognosis but her oncologist noticed that Mrs. J was not getting back to running or her usual activities; she was complaining of poor sleep and seemed irritable. The oncologist had tried multiple benzodiazepines for sleep and nothing seemed to be helping. The amount of narcotics the patient was using for pain relief had remained fairly high. Mrs. J had been followed for several years by a social worker but the oncologist and social worker had never really discussed Mrs. J's care. After the oncologist's several attempts to pursuade the patient to be seen by a psychiatrist, she finally agreed to do so.

The psychiatrist was quite surprised to learn of the patient's long-standing alcohol dependence which had been in remission until the time of the cancer diagnosis. The alcohol dependence disorder had not been discussed with the oncologist because the patient did not want to seem weak or dependent in the doctor's eyes. The social worker had not realized that the patient had started drinking again. The use of narcotics by the patient was additive to the alcohol and the patient was feeling overwhelmed and depressed.

In this case, the oncologist was well meaning in prescribing narcotics to this patient. The patient had been through 12-step programs and viewed any "mind-altering" drug as fostering her addictive problems. At the beginning of her cancer diagnosis and treatment, Mrs. J started feeling depressed and worried about the future. Once the narcotics were prescribed and she started using them regularly, Mrs. J began to lose her confidence and control over her alcohol dependence and resumed using alcohol. The oncologist did not ask about a history of alcohol or substance abuse and the patient did not tell.

The meaning for this patient of the use of narcotics was quite significant and symbolic. It was not simply a way to control pain but rather a recrudescence of a long-standing dependence on oral agents to help control problems in her life. The narcotics as well as the cancer were symbolic of long-standing dependence troubles. Mrs. J was ashamed and humiliated by her alcoholism and therefore tried to withhold very crucial information from her doctor. She also felt that she could combat the problem herself and was frightened of having to enter another alcohol and drug rehabilitation program. Thus, she withheld the information from the social worker.

Patients with drug and alcohol problems often have difficulties with certain types of medication and therefore it is crucial for all clinicians to take a good history at the initial time of treatment as well as throughout the course of care. It is also imperative that the various clinicians involved in management of a patient, especially those patients with drug and alcohol problems, communicate with one another. In Mrs. J's case, had the social worker and oncologist discussed their care of Mrs. J, the history of alcohol dependence and the current signs of alcohol use might have been uncovered.

Specific Diagnostic Issue: Schizophrenia

Another diagnostic disorder where medications have significant meaning is schizophrenia. In this disorder, patients often do not have the ability to tolerate close relationships. In the paranoid type, patients are frequently afraid of taking medications of any type (Winer & Andriukatis, 1989). Patients worry about being poisoned; taking more medication than is needed, and having severe side effects that will affect their weight, sexuality, and ability to think and function. Forming a close bond with a clinician often takes years. In the current health care environment, to sustain a relationship that can provide continuity of care is especially difficult. Patients with schizophrenia may resist change and new medications are often viewed with suspicion and mistrust.

Case 9

Mr. K was a 49-year-old single male who carried the diagnosis of paranoid schizophrenia. He had had two previous psychiatric hospitalizations and was currently being followed at the Community Mental Health Center. His case workers changed almost every 6 months, as did the psychiatrist. Mr. K did not trust his social worker or doctor. He often dropped out of treatment for months and would resurface only when he was in severe psychiatric distress—very paranoid, fearful, and thinking about harming himself. His psychiatrist noted Mr. K's lack of compliance with medications and his inability to keep his clinic appointments and offered monthly injections of haloperidol decanoate. Mr. K viewed this as an aggressive measure and reinforced his paranoid feelings of his doctors wanting to subdue and hurt him. He never returned for follow-up treatment.

While the clinic psychiatrist and social worker were trying to be helpful to Mr. K, he instead viewed their assessment of further treatment and intramuscular decanoate injections as hostile and aggressive. The comments about his noncompliance were taken as harsh criticisms. Instead of trying to ascertain why he wouldn't come for treatments, Mr. K's paranoid fears and thoughts were used to condemn him. Mr. K didn't feel as if he could explain what his problems were—he himself didn't understand. It just seemed to him that the clinic staff was angry at him and therefore wanted to hurt him. He felt he would be better off not returning and just going to the hospital emergency room if he got into serious trouble.

It is unclear from this vignette whether the psychiatrist ever realized what the problem was in the patient not returning for follow-up. Most likely, the patient was blamed and Mr. K's lack of follow-up was offered as evidence of his noncompliance. Issues surrounding the miscommunication in the doctor-patient relationship probably never arose.

While there has been a lot of literature on the subject of forging a positive psychotherapeutic relationship with patients with schizophrenia, it is probably more difficult than ever in today's clinical care climate to be able to attend to all the multiple issues necessary with such patients. There are in general fewer resources and services available for the seriously and chronically mentally ill. There is not a very good system of following up with patients who refuse or don't want treatment. Patients are

TABLE 7.4. Suggestions for Fostering the Doctor-Patient Relationship with Patients with Schizophrenia Treated in a Community Mental Health Center

---

- Doctors and clinic staff need to *review the stability of the relationships* the patients have with them. If too many doctors are being changed for some patients, then this needs to be curtailed. At the very minimum, the topic needs to be discussed with patients.
- Think carefully when *medications are proposed to be changed* and discuss the various meanings this could have for patients.
- Try to *give patients choices* in the medications they need to be on.
- Have a *good follow-up plan* if patients don't show for appointments. The psychiatrist needs to get involved in the follow-up plan.
- *Doctors should try to spend more time,* not less, with patients who are not complying with their treatment. The clinic schedule needs to factor in such problems when apportioning time for patients who have a history of adherence problems.

---

refused inpatient hospitalizations except for the most acute problems and have shorter stays even when hospitalized—less of an opportunity for an entire team to take care of the multiple needs of patients (housing; transportation; job and vocational problems; family issues; medication stabilization).

Time is a key problem. With so many patients followed at community mental health centers, physicians usually see patients very infrequently, often just for medication checks. Other professionals—nurses, social workers, counselors—see the patients more regularly. The bond between doctor and patient is therefore not frequently pursued. It is no wonder, therefore, that Mr. K, who hardly knew the psychiatrist, would make a decision not to return to clinic after he was told he would need intramuscular injections. It sounded like a punishment to him.

Some suggestions of ways to avoid such problems are given in Table 7.4.

CLINICAL SETTINGS THAT FOSTER COMPLICATIONS

There are settings of care that promote problems with doctor-patient relationships (McNutt et al., 1987). For example, some hospitals and insurance systems have doctors who are "hospitalists" (who only see those patients in the hospital) and "generalists" (psychiatrists who follow patients in the outpatient setting).

Case 10

Ms. L, a 16-year-old junior at boarding school, being treated for bulimia nervosa, has returned early from her winter break. Things did not go well at home with her parents. She argued continually with her parents and had felt suicidal.

Prior to winter break, she and her psychiatrist had discussed issues that might come up at home. The patient was thinking about not even going home but her psychiatrist encouraged her to do so—the dormitory would be empty; her parents would have been quite angry and disappointed; and the psychiatrist was not going to be in town.

When Ms. L returned early, she called the psychiatrist. Ms. L left a very tearful, angry message on the answering machine. The psychiatrist requested that Ms. L go to the emergency room and be hospitalized. The psychiatrist did not provide care in the hospital; other members of the HMO psychiatric staff served that function. Much of the focus of the hospitalization was about Ms. L's parents but also about her feelings of abandonment by the psychiatrist.

There are also settings—such as partial hospital programs, community mental health centers, inpatient settings, substance abuse programs—where patients are treated by teams of professionals. Depending on the particular issue (detoxification; job and vocational skills and placement; occupational therapy; medication management; housing and transportation; family problems; etc.), the role of the doctor may or may not be as critical as the role of others on the team.

Patients benefit from the multispecialty nature of such settings and often need the services of a wide and diverse group of professionals. There is a diminution, moreover, in such settings of the role and importance of the doctor-patient relationship. When problems arise, it is sometimes not the doctor that the patient calls first.

It is important, however, for the doctor to understand his or her role, liability, and responsibility for the patient in such settings. The doctor must determine if he or she is in fact in charge of the patient through all phases of care, not just the particular ones he or she is directly providing for the patient. If the doctor is in fact responsible, there needs to be excellent communication processes between the staff and the patient and doctor and frequent and regular contacts between the doctor and the patient.

CONCLUSION

The meaning of medications to patients and their families is complex. The roots have to do with the way illness is understood and perceived. As noted in Chapter 1, many physicians are using terms such as "chemical imbalance" or problems in "brain chemistry" to describe the need for psychotropic medications. While some patients feel relieved that their problems are caused by a brain disorder or biological/physiological disease process and need to take medications, others are frightened, stigmatized, and feel even more helpless, and are angry that they don't have control (Carli, 1999).

The meaning that patients ascribe to medications is quite personal and often has to do with the way medications were discussed by their families; educational background and knowledge about pharmaceuticals and disease processes; transferential feelings toward doctors; individual histories with various medications; what patients know of their family members and friends' psychiatric histories and outcomes; cultural influences; and impact of the media. Patients have certain expectations of medications and psychiatric care based on some of the above factors and too often such issues are not discussed.

A framework, therefore, for understanding the patient and the meaning of medications is sometimes not well understood by clinicians and leads to problems and difficulties. Much in the previous chapters addresses such factors—why some patients have difficulty trusting doctors who are prescribing medication; why there are often adherence issues in following a drug regimen; and the transferential and countertransferential feelings that can influence whether the patient is receiving psychotropic medication and from whom (PCP, psychiatrist, social worker making the referral, etc.).

Further, all clinicians value medications in various ways and it is important to understand such differences. If a social worker refers a patient to a psychiatrist believing in a positive way that a psychotropic medication could assist the therapy, then that could be a helpful referral; if a patient in a capitated system asks her begrudging primary care physician for a referral to a psychiatrist for medication, then the outcome for that patient could obviously be quite different.

This chapter focused on several complex types of clinical situations where the manifest issue is medication but the latent issues relate to complicated dynamic problems. It hopefully helped to embellish some of the case vignettes provided throughout the book and gave clinical insights into the complexity of the psychotherapy of medication. Fundamentally, treatment must be based on sound clinical judgment, assessment of what is occurring in the doctor-patient relationship, and the meaning of medication to the patient, family, and clinicians. The chapter could not be exhaustive since the types of difficult cases abound but rather should be suggestive of the complexity of the issues surrounding the provision of medication. We hope that the case examples provided a stimulus for further discussion and understanding.

References

Adelman, S.A. (1985). Pills as transitional objects: A dynamic understanding of the use of medication in psychotherapy. *Psychiatry, 48,* 246–253.

American Psychiatric Association. (1980a). *Diagnostic and statistical manual of mental disorders* (3rd ed.). Washington, DC: Author.

American Psychiatric Association. (1980b). Guidelines for psychiatrists in consultative, supervisory, or collaborative relationships with nonmedical therapists. *American Journal of Psychiatry, 137,* 1489–1491.

American Psychiatric Association. (1994). *Diagnostic and statistical manual of mental disorders* (4th ed.). Washington, DC: Author.

American Psychiatric Association. (1995). *Principles of medical ethics with annotations especially applicable to psychiatry* (p. 8). Washington, DC: Author.

Anonymous. (1981). What should we tell patients about their medicines? *Drug Therapy Bulletin, 19,* 74.

Appelbaum, P.S. (1991). General guidelines for psychiatrists who prescribe medications for patients treated by nonmedical psychotherapists. *Hospital and Community Psychiatry, 42,* 281–282.

Balon, R. (1999). Positive aspects of collaborative treatment. In M.B. Riba & R. Balon (Eds), *Psychopharmacology and psychotherapy: A collaborative approach* (pp. 1–31). Washington, DC: American Psychiatric Press.

Bassuk, E., & Schoonover, S. (1978). Rampant dental caries in the treatment of depression. *Journal of Clinical Psychiatry, 39,* 163–165.

Bersani, L. (1986). *The Freudian body: Psychoanalysis and art.* New York: Columbia University Press.

Blackwell, B. (1976). Treatment adherence. *British Journal of Psychiatry 129,* 513–531.

References

Book, H.E. (1987). Some psychodynamics of non-compliance. *Canadian Journal of Psychiatry, 32,* 115–117.

Brouceck, F., & Ricci, W. (1998). Self-disclosure of self presence? *Bulletin of the Menninger Clinic, 26*(4), 427–438.

Brown, W.A. (1998). The placebo effect. *Scientific American, 278,* 107–116.

Butler, C., Rollnick, S., & Stott, N. (1996). The practitioner, the patient and resistance to change: Recent ideas on compliance. *Canadian Medical Association Journal, 154,* 1357–1362.

Carli, T. (1999). The psychologically informed psychopharmacologist. In M. B. Riba & R. Balon (Eds.), *Psychopharmacology and psychotherapy: A collaborative approach* (pp. 179–196). Washington, DC: American Psychiatric Press.

Chen, A. (1991). Noncompliance in community psychiatry: A review of clinical interventions. *Hospital and Community Psychiatry, 42,* 282–287.

Chiles, J.A., Carlin, A.S., Benjamin, G.A.H., et al. (1991). A physician, a nonmedical psychotherapist, and a patient: The pharmacotherapy-psychotherapy triangle. In B.D. Beitman & G.D. Klerman (Eds.), *Integrating pharmacotherapy and psychotherapy* (pp. 105–118). Washington, DC: American Psychiatric Press.

Crits-Christoph, P. et al. (1993). The accuracy of the therapist's interpretations and the development of the therapeutic alliance. *Psychotherapy Research, 3* 25–35.

Daley, D.C., Salloum, I.M., Zuckoff, A., et al. (1998). Increasing treatment adherence among outpatients with depression and cocaine dependence: Results of a pilot study. *American Journal of Psychiatry, 155,* 1611–1613.

Dewan, M.J. (1992). Adding medications to ongoing psychotherapy: Indications and pitfalls. *American Journal of Psychotherapy, 46* 102–110.

Docherty, J.P., Marder, S.R., Van Kammen, D.P., et al. (1977). Psychotherapy and pharmacotherapy: Conceptual lenses. *American Journal of Psychiatry, 134,* 529–533.

Eisenthal, S., Koopman, C., & Lazare, A. (1983). Process analysis of two dimensions of the negotiated approach in relation to satisfaction in the initial interview. *Jouranl of Nervous and Mental Disease, 171,* 49–54.

Fairman, K.A., Drevets, W.C., Kreisman, J.J., et al. (1998). Course of antidepressant treatment, drug type, and prescriber's specialty. *Psychiatric Services, 49,* 1180–1186.

Feighner, J.P. (1999). Mechanism of action of antidepressant medications. *Journal of Clinical Psychiatry, 60*(Suppl. 4), 4–13.

Fisher, R., & Ury, W. (1981). *Getting to yes.* Boston: Houghton Mifflin.

Freud, S. (1913). Further recommendations on the technique of psychoanalysis: On beginning treatment. In J. Strachey (Ed. and Trans.), *The standard edition of the complete psychological works of Sigmund Freud* (Vol. XXII). London: Hogarth Press (1953–1964).

Gabbard, G. (Ed.). (1999). *Countertransference issues in psychiatric treatment.* Washington, DC: American Psychiatric Association Press.

Gabbard, G.O., & Wilkinson, S.M. (1994). *Management of countertransference with borderline patients.* Washington, DC: American Psychiatric Press.

Gardner, C.S., Holzman, S.T. (1983). Interdisciplinary collaboration: Psychiatric medical backup in the outpatient clinic. *Psychiatric Quarterly, 55*(4), 253–260.

Gitlin, M.J., Cochran, S.D., & Jamison K.R. (1989). Maintenance lithium treatment: Side effects and compliance. *Journal of Clinical Psychology, 50,* 127–31.

Goldhamer, P.M. (1983). Psychotherapy and pharmacotherapy: The challenge of integration. *Canadian Journal of Psychiatry, 28,* 173–77.

Gove, P.B. (Ed.). (1986). *Webster's third new international dictionary of the English language unabridged.* Springfield, MA: Merriam-Webster.

Gross-Doehrman, M.J. (1976). Parallel processes in supervision and psychotherapy. *Bulletin of the Menninger Clinic, 40*(1), 1–104.

Gunderson, J.G. (1978). Defining the therapeutic processes in psychiatric milieus. *Psychiatry: Journal for the Study of Interpersonal Processes, 41,* 327–335.

Healy, D. (1997). *The antidepressant era.* Cambridge, MA: Harvard University Press.

Imhoff, J., Altman, R., & Katz, J. (1998). The relationship between psychiatrist and prescribing psychotherapist: Some considerations. *American Jouranl of Psychotherapy, 52:3* 261–272.

Jameson, K. (1995). *An unquiet mind: A memoir of moods and madness.* New York: Knopf.

Kane, B., & Sands, D.Z. (1998). Guideline for the clinical use of electronic mail with patients. *Journal of the American Medical Informatics Association, 5,* 104–111.

Kaplan, H.I., & Sadock. B.J. (1989). *Comprehensive textbook of psychiatry* (6th ed.). Baltimore: Williams & Wilkins.

Kendler, K.S., Karkowski, L.M., & Prescott, C.A. (1999). Causal relationship between stressful life events and the onset of major depression. *American Journal of Psychiatry, 156,* 837–841.

Koenigsberg, H.W. (1991). Borderline personality disorder. In B.D. Beitman & G.L. Klerman (Eds.), *Integrating pharmacotherapy and psychotherapy* (pp. 271–290). Washington, DC: American Psychiatric Press.

Kohut, H. (1968). The psychoanalytic treatment of narcissistic personality disorders. *Psychoanalytic Study of the Child, 23,* 86–113.

Kubie, L.S. (1971). The retreat from patients: An unanticipated penalty of the full-time system. *Archives of General Psychiatry, 24,* 98–106.

Lazarus, A. (1995). The role of primary care physicians in managed mental health care. *Psychiatric Services, 46,* 343–345.

Luborsky, L. et al. (1985). Therapist's success and its determinates. *Archives of General Psychiatry, 42,* 602–611.

MacKinnon, R.A., & Michels, R. (1971). *The psychiatric interview in clinical practice*. Philadelphia: Saunders.

Magnavita, J.J. (1993). The evolution of short term dynamic psychotherapy: Treatment of the future? *Professional Psychology: Research and Practice, 24,* 360–365.

Main, T.F. (1957). The ailment. *British Journal of Medical Psychology, 30,* 129–145.

Maltsberger, J.T., & Buie, D.H. (1974). Countertransference hate in the treatment of suicidal patients. *Archives of General Psychiatry, 30,* 633–635.

Marziali, E., Marmar, C., & Krupknick, J. (1981). Therapeutic alliance scales: Development and relationship to psychotherapy outcome. *American Journal of Psychotherapy, 138,* 361–364.

McNutt, E.R., Severino, S.K., & Schomer, J. (1987). Dilemmas in interdisciplinary outpatient care: An approach towards their amelioration. *Journal of Psychiatric Education, 11,* 59–65.

Melfi, C.A., Chawla, A.J., Croghan, T.W., et al. (1998). The effects of adherence to antidepressant treatment guidelines on relapse and recurrence of depression. *Archives of General Psychiatry, 55,* 1128–1132.

Metzl, J.M. (2000). *Signifying medications in Thom Jones's "Superman, My Son": Teaching literature and medicine* (the MLA Approaches to Teaching series). New York: MLA Press.

Morgan, R., Luborsky, L., Crits-Christoph, P., et al. (1982). Predicting the outcomes of psychotherapy by the Penn Helping Alliance Rating Method. *Archives of General Psychiatry, 39,* 397–402.

Noorily, S.H., Hantler, C.B., & Sako, E.Y. (1997). Monoamine oxidase inhibitors and cardiac anesthesia revisited. *Southern Medical Journal, 90,* 836–838.

Owen, R.R., Fischer, E.P., Booth, B.M., et al. (1996). Medication noncompliance and substance abuse among patients with schizophrenia. *Psychatric Services, 47,* 853–858.

Parens, E. (1998, Jan./Feb.) Is better always good? The enhancement project. *Hastings Center Report, 28*(1), 24B–S15.

Reiss, D., Plomin, R., & Hetherington, E.M. (1991). Genetics and psychiatry: An unheralded window on the environment. *American Journal of Psychiatry, 148,* 283–291.

Remick, R.A. (1988). Anticholinergic side effects of tricyclic antidepressants and their management. *Progress in Neuro-Psychopharmacology and Biological Psychiatry, 12*(2–3), 225–231.

Riba, M.R., & Balon, R. (Eds.). (1999). *Psychopharmacology and psychotherapy: A collaborative approach.* Washington, DC: American Psychiatric Press.

Rowland, J.H., & Massie, M.J. (1998). Breast cancer. In J.C. Holland (Ed.), *Psychooncology* (pp. 38–401). New York: Oxford University Press.

Rudd, P. (1979). In search of the gold standard for compliance measurement. *Archives of Internal Medicine, 139,* 627.

References

Schiffman, S. (1999). *The 25 sales habits of highly successful salespeople* (2nd ed.). Holbrook, MA: Bob Adams.

Sederer, L.I., Ellison, J.M., Keyes, C. (1998). Guidelines for prescribing psychiatrists in consultative, collaborative, and supervisory relationships. *Psychiatric Services, 49,* 1197–1202.

Silk, K.R. (1999). Collaborative treatment for patients with personality disorders. In M. B. Riba & R. Balon (Eds.), *Psychopharmacology and psychotherapy: A collaborative approach.* Washington, DC: American Psychiatric Press.

Smith, J. (1989). Some dimensions of transference in combined treatment. In J.M. Ellison (Ed.), *The psychotherapist's guide to pharmacotherapy* (pp. 79–95). Chicago: Year Book Medical Publishers.

Smith, R. (1996). *The patient's story.* Boston: Little, Brown.

Spitzer, R.L., Williams, J.B., Kroenke, K., Linzer, M., deGruy, F.V. III, Hahn, S.R., Brody, D., & Johnson, J.G. (1994). Utility of a new procedure for diagnosing mental disorders in primary care. The PRIME-MD 1000. *Journal of the American Medical Association, 272*(22) 1749–1756.

Steffens, D.C., Krishnan, K.R., & Helms, M.J. (1997). Are SSRIs better than TCAs? Comparison of SSRIs and TCAs: A meta-analysis. *Depression and Anxiety, 6*(1), 10–18.

Tanaka, E., & Hisawa S. (1999). Clinically significant pharmacokinetic drug interactions with psychoactive drugs: Antidepressants and antipsychotics and the cytochrome P450 system. *Journal of Clinical Pharmacy and Therapeutics, 24,* 7–16.

Valenstein, M. (1999). Primary care physicians and mental health professionals: models for collaboration. In M.B. Riba & R. Balon (Eds.). *Psychopharmacology and psychotherapy: A collaborative approach* (pp. 325–352). Washington, DC: American Psychiatric Press.

Waldinger, R.J., & Frank, A.F. (1989a). Clinicians' experiences in combining medication and psychotherapy in the treatment of borderline patients. *Hospital and Community Psychiatry, 40,* 712–718.

Waldinger, R.J., & Frank, A.F. (1989b). Transference and the vicissitudes of medication use by borderline patients. *Psychiatry, 52,* 416–427.

Ward, N.G. (1991). Psychosocial approaches to pharmacotherapy. In B.D. Beitman & G.L. Klerman (eds): *Integrating pharmacotherapy and psychotherapy* (pp. 69–104). Washington, DC: American Psychiatric Press.

Warner, L.A., Silk, K., Yeaton, W.H., et al. (1994). Psychiatrists' and patients' views on drug information sources and medication compliance. *Hospital and Community Psychiatry, 45,* 1235–1237.

Weiss, R.D., Greenfield, S.F., Najavits, L.M., et al. Medication compliance among patients with bipolar disorder and substance abuse disorder. *Journal of Clinical Psychology, 59,* 172–174.

Winer, J., & Andriukatis, S. (1989). Interpersonal aspects of initiating pharmacotherapy: How to avoid becoming the patient's feared negative other. *Psychiatric Annals, 19,* 318–323.

Winnicott, D. (1953). Transitional objects and transitional phenomena. *International Journal of Psycho-Analysis, 34,* 89–97.

Woodward, B., Duckworth, K.S., & Gutheil, T.G. (1993). The pharmacotherapist-psychotherapist collaboration. In J.M. Oldham, M.B. Riba, & A. Tasman (Eds.), *American Psychiatric Press review of psychiatry* (Vol. 12, pp. 631–649). Washington, DC: American Psychiatric Press.

Zisook, S., Hammond, R., Jaffe, K., et al. (1978–79). Outpatient requests, initial sessions and attrition. *International Journal of Psychiatry and Medicine, 9,* 339–350.

Zita, J. (1998). *Body talk.* New York: Columbia University Press.

Index